THE BRANEMARK IMPLANT SYSTEM
Clinical and Laboratory Procedures

John Beumer III, D.D.S., M.S.

Professor and Chairman
Removable Prosthodontics
Co-director, UCLA Oral-facial Implant Center
School of Dentistry
University of California, Los Angeles

Steven G. Lewis, D.M.D.

Adjunct Assistant Professor,
Removable Prosthodontics
Co-director, UCLA Oral-facial Implant Center
School of Dentistry
University of California, Los Angeles

Ishiyaku EuroAmerica, Inc.
St. Louis • Tokyo

Book Editor: Gregory Hacke, D.C.

Ishiyaku EuroAmerica, Inc.
716 Hanley Industrial Court, St. Louis, Missouri 63144

Library of Congress Catalogue Number 89-45807

Beumer, John III, D.D.S., M.S.
Lewis, Steven G., D.M.D.
   The Branemark Implant System:
   Clinical and Laboratory Procedures

ISBN 0-912791-62-4

Ishiyaku EuroAmerica, Inc.
St. Louis • Tokyo

Composition by: Characters, Collinsville, Illinois
Printed in the Spain by: Espaxs, S.A. Publicaciones Médicas

DEDICATION

To Jan and Carol

FOREWARD

The edentulous patient – having lost one, several, or all teeth – is looking for a prosthetic substitute that can provide adequate masticatory, phonetic, and esthetic function equal to normal dentition; without jeopardizing remaining teeth or jaw bone in the short or long term perspective.

Osseointegrated titanium fixtures have been shown to provide the necessary retention and stability for artificial teeth as documented in multi-center consecutive clinical studies. A variety of surgical techniques, including grafting procedures, have been developed so that almost every patient, irrespective of defect anatomy, can be provided with anchorage to the edentulous jaw bone.

There has, however, been a definite need for a summarizing review of prosthetic methodology involving presurgical planning of therapy. This review should include careful consideration of treatment alternatives, final clinical results to be expected, and materials and procedures to be used for designing and manufacturing the prosthesis.

Intricate technical details have to be handled in adjusting the prosthesis to structural and functional demands in order to provide the best possible oral and total rehabilitation of the individual patient. These technical details require a broad base of prosthodontic experience in conjunction with creative thinking and an innovative approach, identifying possibilities rather than limitations and obstacles.

Based on their own clinical experience with osseointegration in oral and maxillofacial rehabilitation, Dr. John Beumer and Dr. Steven Lewis have written a book that will provide the practitioner with the information necessary to advise patients about realistic treatment alternatives. They have also provided the surgeon with valuable information on how to place the fixtures to make them most useful for the prosthodontist and beneficial for the patient. But certainly the foremost aim of the book is to describe clinically proven prosthetic procedures that can be applied in cases of different degrees and anatomical types of edentulism, providing predictable and lasting return to a fixed dentition.

The book is characterized by attention to precision in all details of component selection, how to join them to a functioning prosthesis, and how to successively perform adjustments in order to make the tissue – integrated prosthesis an accepted, well functioning part of the patient's body. It was necessary for a book of this kind to be written, and it was important that prosthodontists of Dr. Beumer's and Dr. Lewis' capacity did it.

Per-Ingvar Brånemark
M.D., Ph.D., O.Dhc.

PREFACE

Rehabilitation of patients rendered edentulous has always been a difficult challenge. Because of the work of Dr. P.I. Branemark, an implant system has been developed which can restore these patients to near normal function in a highly predictable fashion. In partially edentulous patients this new system of osseointegrated implants is beginning to be employed, and although longitudinal data is not yet available, the initial results look promising in selected patients. The purpose of this atlas is to provide a detailed description of the method used to design and fabricate prosthetic restorations using the implant system developed by Dr. P.I. Branemark.

Modern oral implantology truly has become multidisciplinary in nature, requiring that all members of the team – surgeon, restorative dentist, and dental laboratory technician – be familiar with the role and responsibilities of their fellows. Here at UCLA we have proceeded in this fashion from the time our implant program was initiated, and as a result there have been few complications or necessary design compromises associated with the definitive treatment offered the patient. Obviously, best results are achieved when the definitive restorative plan has been established before the implants are surgically placed.

Compiling an atlas of this size and scope required the efforts of many talented and dedicated individuals. Most important are the fellow members of our UCLA Oral-facial implant team – Dr. Peter Moy, Dr. E. B. Kenney, Dr. Ray Lee, Dr. Michael Hamada, and Dr. Michael Engelman. Drs. Hamada, Lee, and Engleman provided the illustrations for many of the figures in this book. We are also indebted to Wyn Hornberg, Sean Avera, and Gary Nunokawa because of their superb dental laboratory support. The contribution of Wynn Hornberg is particularly noteworty, for he is the co-inventor of the ''UCLA'' abutment. Special thanks are given to Dr. Fred Herzberg for his editorial assistance and Mickey Stern for typing the manuscript.

John Beumer III, D.D.S., M.S.
Steven G. Lewis, D.M.D.

TABLE OF CONTENTS

CHAPTER 1

Factors Important in Achieving and Maintaining Osseointegration

INTRODUCTION

Osseointegration, as defined by Per-Ingvar Branemark, is a "direct structural and functional connection between ordered, living bone and the surface of a load-carrying implant." Through three decades of research and development, including both laboratory and clinical studies, Branemark and his colleagues have provided us with an implant system that can replace lost natural teeth by tissue-integrated tooth root analogues. The initial high levels of success reported by these Swedish researchers are now being achieved by dentists throughout the world. Osseointegration has revolutionized the way in which we treat edentulous and partially edentulous patients and, as time goes on, will play a major role in virtually all aspects of dental medicine. This chapter will discuss the important biologic factors which enable pure titanium implant fixtures to achieve a state of osseointegration with the surrounding bone.

DEFINITION

Osseointegration is defined as a "direct structural and functional connection between ordered, living bone and the surface of a load-carrying implant" (Branemark, 1985). The basic concepts evolved from a series of experiments begun in the early 1960s that were aimed at studying the response of bone marrow to various trauma and clinical procedures. (Professor Per-Ingvar Branemark is shown in Fig. 1-1.)

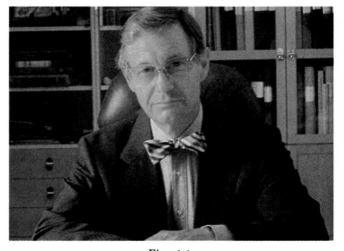

Fig. 1-1

1

BASIC RESEARCH: BONE INTERFACE

Bone is an extremely dynamic tissue that is responsible for a number of vital body functions. In the early 1960s, P.I. Branemark and his colleagues began studying bone with in vivo light microscopy. To do so, they fabricated a metal chamber and embedded it in the tibia of a rabbit. For reasons not entirely clear, pure titanium was the metal chosen. A diagrammatic representation of the chamber is shown. *(Redrawn from T. Albrektsson, J. Prosth. Dent. 50:255-261, 1983.)*

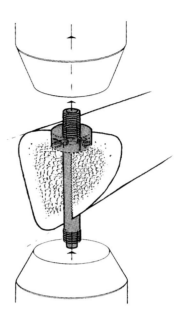

Fig. 1-2

The actual titanium chamber embedded in the rabbit tibia is shown here *(Branemark, 1985)*. The initial studies focused on the functional relationships between bone marrow and bone tissues during regeneration of traumatically induced bony defects. When the researchers attempted to remove the titanium chamber from the subject animal, an important observation was made; the metal optical chamber had become incorporated within the bone and the calcified bony tissue was closely adherent to the tiniest irregularities of the titanium surface. *(From Branemark, P.I., et al., Tissue-Integrated Prostheses, Quintessence Publishing Co., Chicago, Ill., 1985.)*

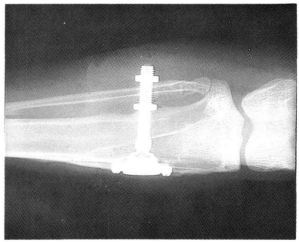

Fig. 1-3

As a consequence of this observation, experiments were conducted which culminated in the development of a screw shaped titanium implant fixture *(Branemark, P.I. 1983)*. Note the adaptation of the bone at the bone site to the surface configuration of the implant fixture. *(From Branemark, P.I., Tissue Integrated Prostheses, Quintessence Publishing Co., Chicago, Ill., 1985.)*

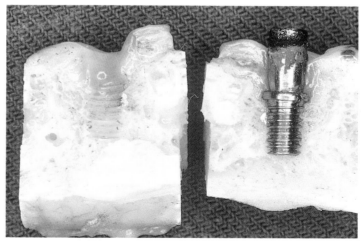

Fig. 1-4

Long term animal studies were then conducted. Implant fixtures of pure titanium were placed in the jaw bones of mongrel dogs, and fixed partial dentures were fabricated and allowed to function for as long as 10 years *(Branemark, P.I. 1983)*. A roentgenogram (Fig. 1-5,A) of such an implant supported fixed partial denture (Fig. 1-5,B) four years following insertion is shown. Note the absence of bone resorption around the implant fixtures *(From Branemark, P:I., Scand. J. Plast. Reconstr. Surg. 3:81-100, 1969.)*

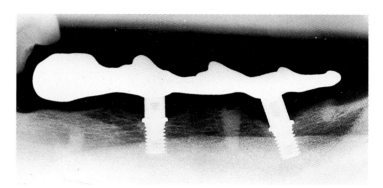

Fig. 1-5,A

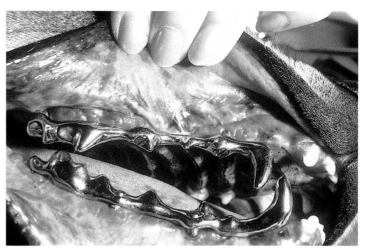

Fig. 1-5,B

Specimens obtained from these animals were examined with light microscopy and revealed a very close adaptation between the surface of the titanium implant fixture and the adjacent bone. Of note was the absence of a fibrous connective tissue interface between the titanium and bone *(courtesy P.I. Branemark).*

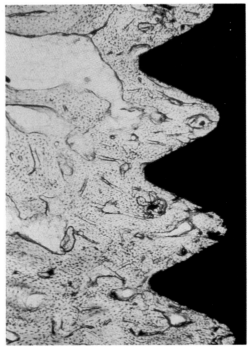

Fig. 1-6

Further animal studies using the scanning electron microscope also revealed that a close association between titanium and bone can be achieved. These experiments indicated that the bone was not separated from the titanium surface by a fibrous connective tissue membrane. Collagen bundles were observed, but were always separated by a proteoglycan layer, a portion of which was calcified *(Hansson, H-A, et al., 1983).* Fig. 1-7. Titanium Bone Interface with Scanning Electrons Microscopy.

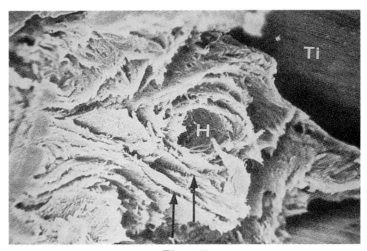

Fig. 1-7

Bone has an unusual affinity for titanium. In an experiment conducted at UCLA, tissue culture colonies of bone cells have readily proliferated and calcified on pure titanium foil (Fig. 1-8), whereas on chrome cobalt alloy foil similar bone cell colonies were rarely seen. Bone cell colonies did not grow with the same abundance on titanium alloy foil (Kenney, 1987).

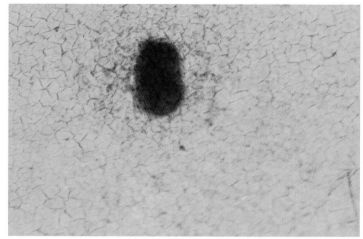

Fig. 1-8

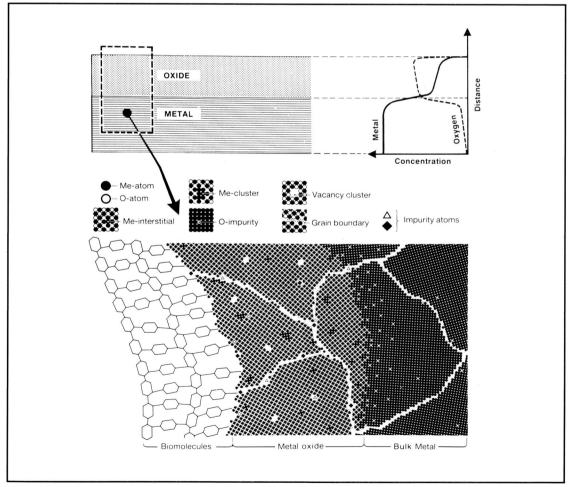

Fig. 1-9

The unique properties of titanium and the oxide layer that forms on its surface are in part responsible for its ability to obtain and maintain a state of osseointegration. It has been speculated that there are a number of types of bonding which unite the biomolecules to the titanium oxide layer when the surface is properly treated and prepared. These include van der Waals bonding, hydrogen bonding, and local chemical bonds. The specific nature of these biomolecular relationships, however, has yet to be determined. *(Branemark, P.I., et al. Tissue Integrated Prostheses, Quintessence Publishing Co., Chicago, Ill., 1985.)* Figure 1-9 shows a schematic drawing of the surface interaction.

EFFECT OF CLINICAL PROCEDURES ON OSSEOINTEGRATION

Careful preparation of the recipient bone site is critical to consistently obtaining a state of osseointegration between implant fixture and bone. During surgery, bone temperatures above 47° centigrade lead to impaired healing and increased likelihood of a connective tissue interface forming between implant fixture and bone *(Eriksson A.R. and Albrektsson, T., 1983)*. The implant site is being tapped to receive a "Branemark" implant. The rotary instrument is programmed not to exceed 15 revolutions per minute.

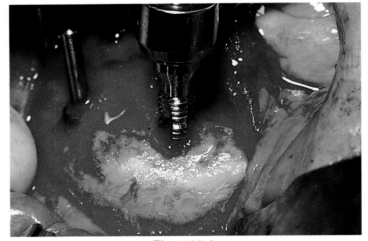

Fig. 1-10,A

Figure 1-10,B shows the completed tapped bone site.

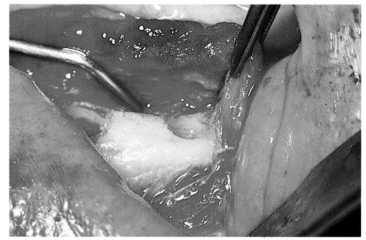

Fig. 1-10,B

Loading an implant prematurely may result in unwanted mobility of the implant fixture, impairing the mechanisms of bone repair at the bone implant interface and resulting in fibrous connective tissue encapsulation of the implant fixture. In addition, sufficient time must be allowed for the bone to heal and grow against the microarchitecture of the implant surface. In the mandible, a minimum of four months is required, while in the maxilla a minimum of six months is necessary. Regular follow-up examinations are required in order to discover and manage premature exposures of the implant fixtures through the oral mucosa. In this patient the top of some of the implant fixtures can be seen through the oral mucosa.

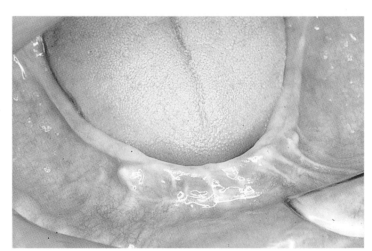

Fig. 1-11

If the prescribed procedures are not carefully followed, a fibrous connective tissue interface develops (Fig. 1-12,A) as opposed to direct bone contact between bone and titanium implant surfaces (Fig. 1-12,B) (Branemark et al., 1985).

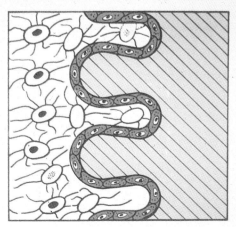

Fig. 1-12,A

The latter has proven to be favored over the former and appears to be superior with respect to long term clinical outcomes in human patients.

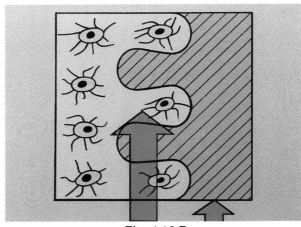

Fig. 1-12,B

EPITHELIAL INTERFACE

Human specimen and animal studies appear to indicate that oral epithelium can effect a close association and adherence with a variety of materials piercing it, including teeth and dental implants. Epithelial cells in close association with dental implants adhere to these surfaces by secreting a basal lamina and forming hemidesmosomes *(Cate, A.R. 1985)*. If the implant pierces a bed of keratinized attached mucosa, well organized circumimplant collagen fibers form a network around the implant and bring the epithelium of the oral mucosa into close approximation with the implant surface, allowing the formation of a quasi "epithelial attachment" *(from Branemark, P.I., Tissue Integrated Prostheses, Quintessence, Chicago, Ill., 1983).*

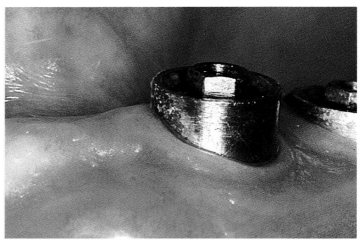

Fig. 1-13

Apical growth of epithelium in natural dentition is usually preceded by inflammation and subsequent breakdown of the underlying connective tissue adjacent to the tooth. It seems evident that in the case of osseointegrated implants, even in the face of inadequate oral hygiene and obvious inflammation associated with the peri-implant submucosal collagenous tissue, apical epithelial migration does not occur. The factors responsible for this phenomenon have not been elucidated. This gingival specimen was taken from tissues adjacent to a "Branemark" implant. Note the absence of apical epithelial migration. *(Courtesy P.I. Branemark)*.

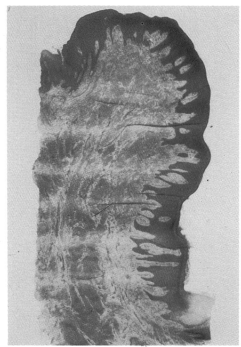

Fig. 1-14

With respect to osseointegrated implants, an entirely different mechanism of attachment is seen. This mechanism is similar to ankylosis, and apparently is responsible for its long-term clinical predictability. Past efforts aimed at creating an implant attachment equivalent to the highly specialized periodontal ligament have resulted in the creation of poorly differentiated fibrous connective interfaces bearing little resemblance to the periodontium and predisposing to connective tissue breakdown and epithelial migration.

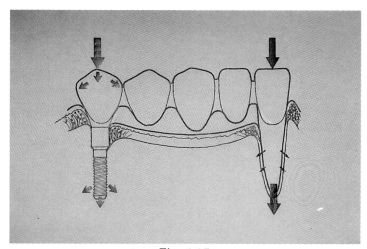

Fig. 1-15

DESIGN OF COMPONENTS

The surface of the implant fixture must be free of undesirable contaminants prior to use if optimal results are to be achieved. Careful preparation and handling of implant fixtures during placement will insure consistent results. It has been suggested that specific surface contaminants may impair the initial healing and compromise the degree of osseointegration between bone and implant fixture.

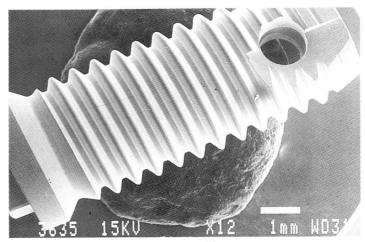

Fig.1-16

After several years of research, initially in dogs and later in humans, a screw design evolved. This design allows for a significant increase in the surface contact areas between the bone and implant fixture. In addition, the screw design distributed the occlusal loads widely to the investing bone, avoiding concentration of stress at undesirable locations. The tips of the screw threads are rounded to avoid concentration of stress at these points.

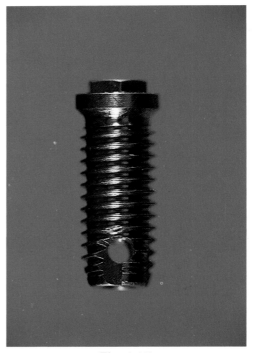

Fig. 1-17

Using photoelastic and finite element analysis, the "Branemark" and other osseointegrated implant designs have been tested extensively. It has been speculated that after loading, inappropriate stress concentration may lead to crestal bone loss around an implant. Indeed, in this other implant design stresses concentrate at specific points, and may be the cause of the rapid crestal bone loss observed upon loading, as reported by Moy (1987). The stress pattern observed with the application of a 40 pound apical load indicates that the "Branemark" implant fixture distributes stresses widely and in an apparently biologically acceptable manner *(Kinni, M. et al., 1987)*.

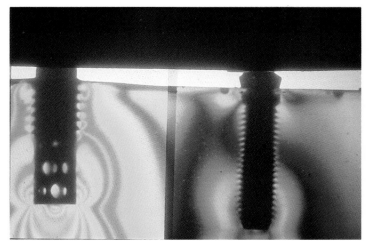

Fig. 1-18

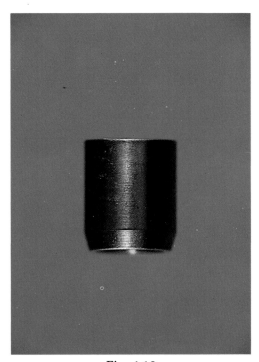

Fig. 1-19

In the "Branemark" design, abutment cylinders connect to the implant fixtures and penetrate the oral mucosa. Lengths from 3 mm to 10 mm are provided to accommodate for the varying thickness of the mucoperiosteum The abutment cylinder is a machined surface of pure titanium.

It is desirable that the abutment cylinders exit the mucosa in a bed of keratinized attached tissue. The abutment cylinder on the left is entirely surrounded by keratinized attached tissue. Note the gingival cuff formed around the cylinder. The labial surface tissue of the abutment on the right consists of unattached tissue, and a similar gingival cuff is lacking. If implants exit in attached mucosal beds, oral hygiene is facilitated and the incidence of soft tissue complications around the abutment cylinder appears to be decreased.

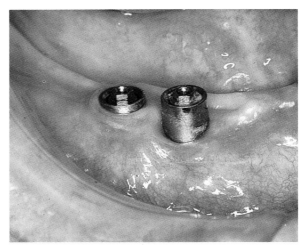

Fig. 1-20

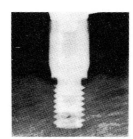 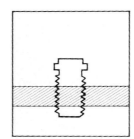 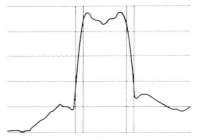

Fig. 1-21,A   Fig. 1-21,B   Fig. 1-21,C

Upon placement of the abutment cylinder, properly executed radiographs can be used to determine if the implant fixtures are indeed osseointegrated. Periapical roentgenograms are obtained using the right angle technique (Fig. 1-20,A). Densitometric analysis of periapical roentgenograms of an osseointegrated implant fixture (Fig. 1-21,B) will indicate increased density (Fig. 1-21,C) of bone adjacent to the fixture, with absence of a soft tissue interface *(courtesy P.I. Branemark)*.

REFERENCES

1. Albrektsson, T.: Direct bone anchorage of dental implants. J. Prosthet. Dent. 50:255-261, 1983.

2. Branemark, P-I., Zarb, H.A. and Albrektsson, T.: Tissue-Integrated Prostheses. Osseointegration in Clinical Dentistry. Quintessence Publishing Co., Inc., Chicago, 1985.

3. Branemark, P-I.: Osseointegration and its experimental background. J. Prosthet. Dent. 50:399-410, 1983.

4. Branemark, P-I.: Intraosseous anchorage of dental prostheses. I. Experimental studies. Scand. J. Plast. Reconstr. Surg. 3:81-100, 1969.

5. Eriksson, A.R. and Albrektsson, T.: Temperature threshold levels for heat-induced bone tissue injury: A vital-microscope study in the rabbit. J. Prosthet. Dent. 50:101-107, 1983.

6. Hansson, H-A., Albrektsson, T. and Branemark, P-I.: Structural aspects of the interface between tissue and titanium implants. J. Prosthet. Dent. 50:108-113, 1983.

7. Kinni, M., Hokama, S.N., Caputo, A.: Force transfer by osseointegration, Int. J. Oral Max Implants. 1:11-14, 1987.

8. Moy, P., Lewis, S., and Beumer, J.: Comparative analysis of one hundred consecutively placed ''Core-Vents'' to one hundred consecutively placed ''Biotes'' implants. Proceedings of Second International Congress on Preprosthetic Surgery (May, 1987).

CHAPTER 2 Patient Selection and Treatment Planning

INTRODUCTION

A number of factors must be considered before selecting a patient for osseointegrated implants. First, the patient must be in reasonable health. The use of these implant systems should probably be avoided in patients with chronic diseases, diabetes and osteoporosis, for example, until appropriate laboratory and clinical studies can be completed. Second, in the healthy patient there must be sufficient amounts of bone at the desired implant sites. The bone must be sufficiently dense at these sites to allow the surgeon to secure appropriate initial anchorage of the implant fixture. Third, it is advisable that the site be covered with some residual keratinized attached tissue. The purpose of this Chapter is to review the physical and anatomic criteria important in patient selection and treatment planning.

RADIOGRAPHIC ANALYSIS (EDENTULOUS PATIENT)

In edentulous and partially edentulous patients, bone quantity and bone quality are two prime factors that are important to consider in patient selection. A panoramic radiograph is the first step in determining the bony nature of the potential implant sites, although definitive determination of the above should not be made with this film. The nature of the cortical and cancellous portion of the bone sites cannot be accurately detected with this method, and there are significant distortions in spatial relationships.

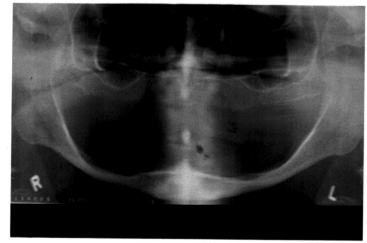

Fig. 2-1

The lateral cephalometric radiograph gives the clinician a good appreciation of the thickness of cortical bone and the amount and nature of cancellous bone at the midline, and is therefore a useful tool in the selection of potential edentulous candidates. Additionally, there is considerably less spatial distoration seen in this view when compared with the panoramic radiograph. The lateral cephalometric radiograph also provides important information in regard to anterior alveolar ridge contour, prominence of the genial tubercle, and jaw relationships.

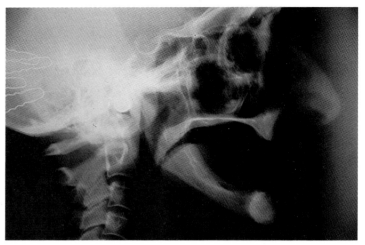

Fig. 2-2

Lekholm and Zarb (1985) have attempted to classify the edentulous mandible and maxilla (Fig. 2-3) as a guide for selection of patients for osseointegrated implants. Their classification system addresses bone morphology (Fig. 2-4,A) and bone density (Fig. 2-4,B). *(Redrawn from Lekholm, and Zarb, G.A. Tissue Integrated Prosthesis, ed. by Branemark, P.I., et al., Quintessence Publishing Co., Chicago, Ill., 1985.)*

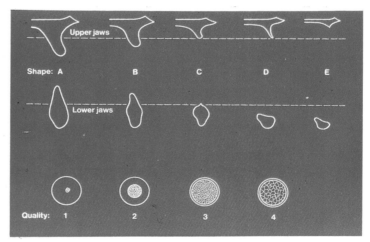

Fig. 2-3

CLASSIFICATION	BONE QUANTITY
A.	Most of the alveolar ridge is present.
B.	Moderate alveolar ridge resorption has occurred.
C.	Advanced alveolar ridge resorption has occurred and only basal bone remains.
D.	Some resorption of the basal bone has taken place.
E.	Extreme resorption of the basal bone has taken place.

(From Lekholm, U., and Zarb, G.A. Tissue Integrated Prosthesis, ed. by Branemark, P.I., et al, Quintessence Publishing Co., Chicago, Ill., 1985.)

Fig. 2-4,A

CLASSIFICATION	BONE QUANTITY
1.	The entire mandible/maxilla is composed of homogenous compact bone.
2.	A thick layer of compact bone surrounds a core of dense trabecular bone.
3.	A thin layer of cortical bone surrounds a core of low density trabecular bone of favorable strength.
4.	A thin layer of cortical bone surrounds a core of low-density trabecular bone.

(Redrawn from Lekholm, and Zarb, G.A. Tissue Integrated Prosthesis, ed. by Branemark, P.I., et al., Quintessence Publishing Co., Chicago, Ill., 1985.)

Fig. 2-4,B

The lateral cephalometric radiograph of this patient indicates category "A" morphology of the mandible in cross section at the midline. In view of the moderate marrow density and relatively thin cortical plate, bone quality would be judged as category "3". This patient would be a reasonably good candidate for osseointegrated implants, all other factors being noncontributory. It may be wise, however, for the surgeon to engage the cortical plate of the inferior border of the mandible in order to enhance initial stabilization of the implant fixtures.

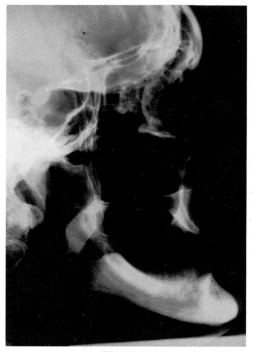

Fig. 2-5

The lateral cephalometric radiograph of this patient indicates a category "A" morphology of the maxilla. However, because of the thin outer layer of cortical bone and the low-density marrow, bone quality is judged as category "4". Great care must be taken in order to achieve solid anchorage of the implant fixture during surgery. In this poor quality bone it is quite easy for the surgeon to over-countersink or strip the threads of the bone site during preparation. In patients with this bone quality, consideration should be given to lengthening the healing time to 8-10 months before performing the Stage II abutment connection (Johanson and Albrektsson, 1987). In our series at UCLA, most of the implant failures have occurred in category "4" (bone quality) maxillae.

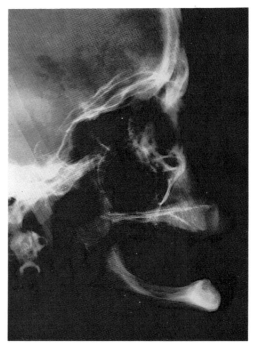

Fig. 2-6

The lateral cephalometric radiograph of this subject indicates a category "D" morphology of the mandible. But, since the entire jaw in cross section appears to be composed of dense homogenous cortical bone, it is judged category "1" in bone quality. Since the mandible is narrow bucco-lingually, the surgeon must take great care in order not to fracture the mandible during implant fixture placement. Since short implants must be used, consideration should be given to placing at least 5 implant fixtures if a fixed bone anchored bridge is planned.

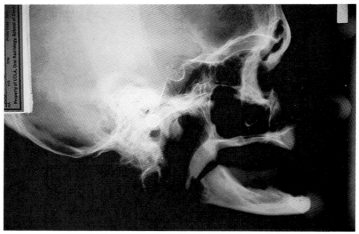

Fig. 2-7

The lateral cephalometric radiograph of this subject demonstrates a category "E" morphology of the maxilla. The resorption process has progressed to where it has affected basalar bone. In most such patients there may only be sufficient bone remaining for two implants—one each in the cuspid area between the anterior extension of the maxillary sinus and the lateral wall of the nose anteriorly. In these instances, autogenous bone grafts may be used to supplement the bone bed.

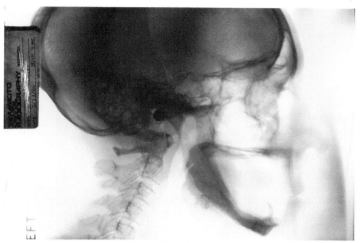

Fig. 2-8

It should be emphasized that the initial successes with the "Branemark" system were achieved in the anterior maxilla and anterior mandible. This panoramic radiograph demonstrates why few patients are candidates for implant placement in the posterior maxilla: 1) in the posterior region, the maxillary sinsuses often extend quite close to the level of the alveolar ridge; 2) in the region just anterior to the sinus, the quantity of bone can be insufficient (at UCLA, most of the failures have been at this site); 3) posterior to the sinus, in the tuberosity region, the bone is of poor quality. Placement of implants in this area is not recommended. The efficacy of the combined sinus lift and bone graft procedure at this site has yet to be determined.

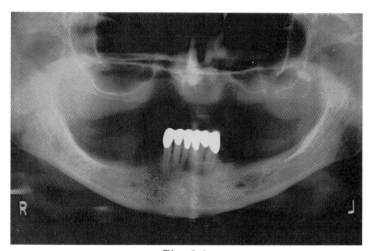

Fig. 2-9

In the posterior mandible, the neuro-vascular bundle is the most important structure limiting implant placement. A minimum of 8 mm of bone between the top of the neurovascular bundle and the aveolar ridge crest is required if a 7 mm implant is to be used. In edentulous patients, we recommend that implants be placed anterior to the mental foramen. There are several reasons for this: 1) 4-6 implants in this region have been found adequate to support a fixed bone anchored bridge designed to restore the posterior occlusion; 2) in patients with category "4" bone quality, the implant fixtures can be made to engage both the inferior and superior cortical plates, thereby enhancing stability of the implant fixture; 3) the mandible flexes posteriorly as much as 1-2 mm upon maximum opening. A full arch rigid fixed partial denture connected to multiple osseointegrated implants posteriorly may precipitate undesirable signs and symptoms due to this flexure and lead to loss of implant fixtures.

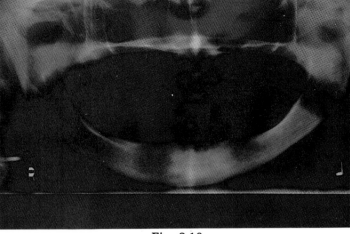

Fig. 2-10

RADIOGRAPHIC ANALYSIS (PARTIALLY EDENTULOUS MANDIBLE)

Osseointegrated implants are now being placed in the posterior mandible in partially edentulous patients (Figs. 2-11, A and B). In these patients, because of the presence of the inferior alveolar nerve, there is generally less bone available. The quality (density) of the posterior mandibular bone site is also inferior to that seen in the edentulous anterior mandible. With only one cortical plate available for engagement, it would appear that the success rates in this region will probably be less than that achieved in the anterior edentulous mandible. Long term data at the present time are not available to indicate the success rates in this region.

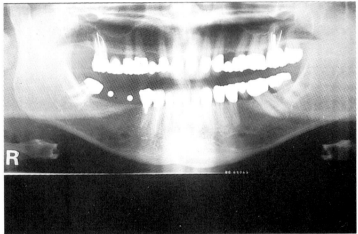

Fig. 2-11,A

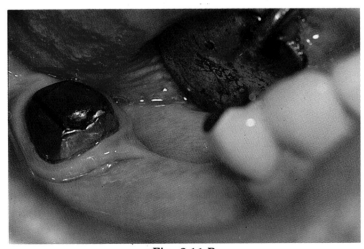

Fig. 2-11,B

When considering a posterior mandibular site for implant fixture placement in a partially edentulous patient, a number of factors must be taken into account:

1. Bone Quality (Fig. 2-12,A)

2. Position of the neurovascular bundle (Fig. 2-12,A)

3. Length of the implants that can be used

4. Size of the edentulous space and the nature of the proposed occlusal loads (Fig. 2-12,B)

It may be desirable to design the implant-supported prosthesis independent of the natural dentition. It is recommended that two or more implants be placed in such edentulous spaces. Where bone is available for only one implant, the implant-supported restoration must be connected to a natural tooth by means of an attachment or a telescopic coping.

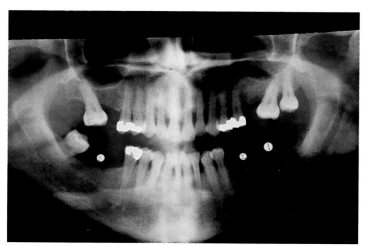

Fig. 2-12,A

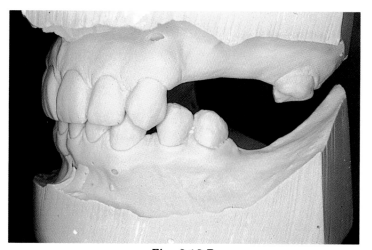

Fig. 2-12,B

The panoramic radiograph is not useful for calculating the precise amount of bone available at the potential implant sites. Since there is little room for error in the posterior mandible, tomographic analysis is necessary. Tomographic projections are shown of the two proposed implant sites noted on the panorex. With this method, precise calculations can be made to determine the amount of bone available, and injury to the inferior alveolar nerve can be avoided.

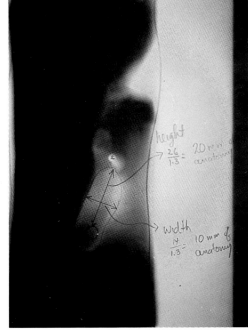

Fig. 2-13

RADIOGRAPHIC ANALYSIS (PARTIALLY EDENTULOUS MAXILLA)

Shown is a panoramic radiograph of a patient edentulous in the posterior maxilla. There is often insufficient bone to receive multiple implants posterior to the cuspid site. In addition, the quality of bone in this region is generally poor. Unless there is sufficient bone to accept at least two 10 mm fixtures in this region, a conventional removable partial denture should be considered.

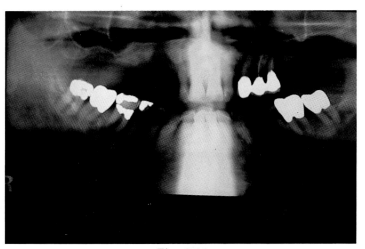

Fig. 2-14

Tomograms (Fig. 2-15,A) of the proposed posterior maxillary sites enable the clinician to visualize the contour of the maxillary sinuses as they extend anteriorly and inferiorly into the maxillary dental alveolus. Computerized axial tomography (Fig. 2-15,B) may also be useful in determining bone morphology at these potential maxillary implant sites. However, its cost limits its usefulness at present. The images obtained can be distorted by existing metallic dental restorations.

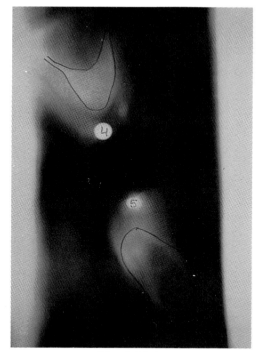

Fig. 2-15,A

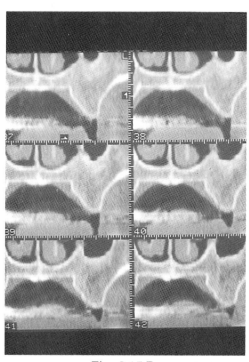

Fig. 2-15,B

In patients edentulous in the anterior maxillary region, the labial-lingual thickness of the alveolus and the extension of the floor of the nose can be appreciated with tomograms or CAT scans. The concavity associated with the incisive fossa and the incisive canal can also be identified with this method.

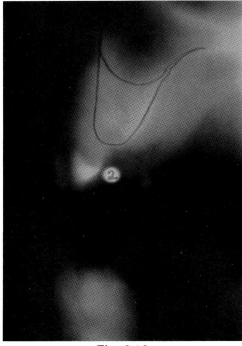

Fig. 2-16

OTHER FACTORS

The panoramic radiograph indicates that recent extractions have been performed on this patient. Six to 12 months of healing are necessary before implants can be placed at these sites. Moderate to severe periodontal bone loss resulting in smaller extraction sites may allow for shorter healing times. At present it is not recommended to place osseointegrated implants into fresh extraction sites.

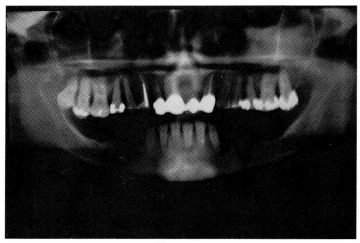

Fig. 2-17

A careful analysis of the soft tissue bed of potential implant sites will avoid undesirable mucosal sequellae following implant placement. At right is a patient with ample attached gingiva remaining (Fig. 2-18,A). If the implants are circumscribed by attached gingiva as they exit the mucosa, a tight gingival cuff will form (Fig. 2-18,B) and oral hygiene and soft tissue maintenance will be achieved more easily.

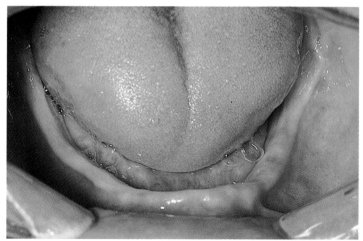

Fig. 2-18,A

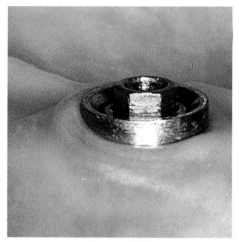

Fig. 2-18,B

Figure 2-19,A shows a patient lacking attached mucosa at the potential implant sites. The tight gingival cuff seen previously is not formed readily (Fig. 2-19,B) and as a consequence, hygiene and gingival maintainence is more difficult. Consideration should be given in some cases to creating an attached keratinized mucosal bed using a free palatal graft. Skin graft vestibuloplasty has also worked effectively in these circumstances. A submucosal resection performed at the time of the second stage surgery can be used to create an attached tissue around the implants.

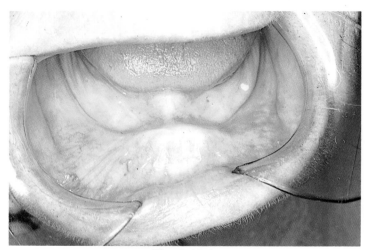

Fig. 2-19,A

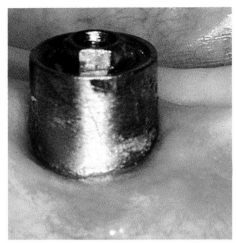

Fig. 2-19,B

This patient presents with a strip of keratinized attached gingiva lingual to the potential implant sites (Fig. 2-20,A). Although far from ideal, a small strip as seen in this patient is sufficient to enable reasonable oral hygiene and maintenance of soft tissue health (Fig. 2-20,B). Palatal graft or skin graft vestibuloplasty is not necessary in most patients such as this one.

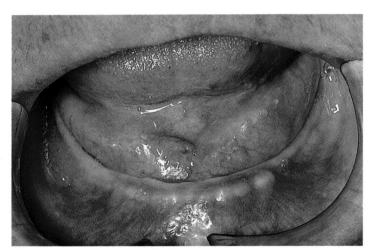

Fig. 2-20,A

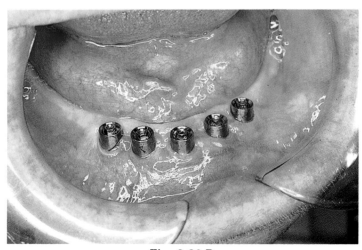

Fig. 2-20,B

High frenum or muscle attachments on either the labial, buccal, or lingual should be excised prior to implant placement if they are adjacent to potential sites. If the soft tissue bed around the implants is excessively mobile, hypertrophy of the mucosa and granulation tissue formation may result.

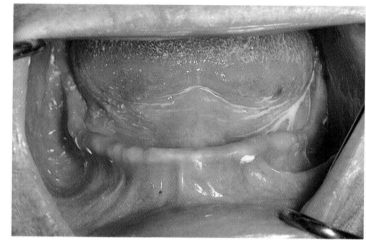

Fig. 2-21

Partially edentulous patients, particularly those who have not worn removable partial dentures, have great amounts of attached mucosa. This makes the soft tissue beds ideal for implant placement.

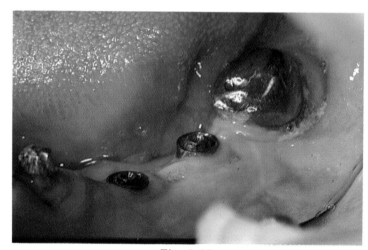

Fig. 2-22

Patients who have worn poorly-adapted and under-extended distal extension removable partial dentures for a prolonged period usually present with significant bone resorption in the posterior edentulous area; there is also loss of some of the attached mucosa. The above combination usually makes them poor candidates for implant placement in the posterior mandible (Figs. 2-23,A and B).

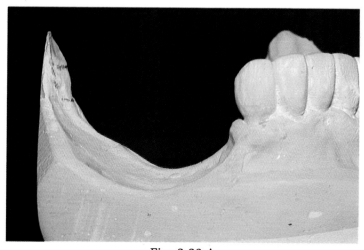

Fig. 2-23,A

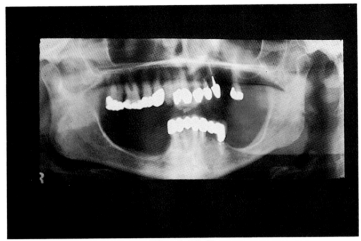

Fig. 2-23,B

Dental compliance is also an important factor to be taken into account when considering a patient for osseointegrated implants. Note the poor oral hygiene around the implants supporting this bone anchored bridge (Fig. 2-24,A).

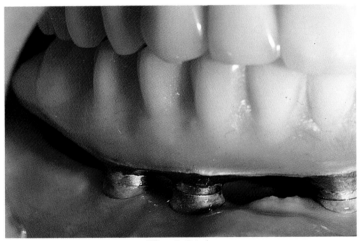

Fig. 2-24,A

Manual dexterity, visual acuity and dental awareness may dictate the nature and design of the implant-supported prosthesis. For example, implants associated with an overdenture (Fig. 2-24,B) are more accessible and thus more easily cleaned by the patient than implants and the exposed undersurfaces of a fixed bone-anchored bridge.

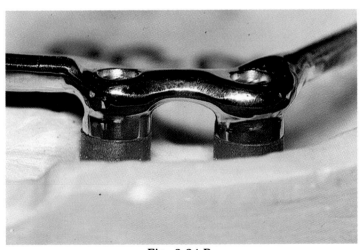

Fig. 2-24,B

REFERENCES

1. Lekholm, U. and Zarb, G.: Patient Selection and Preparation in Tissue Integated Prostheses—Osseointegration in Clinical Dentistry, ed. by Branemark, P-I, G. and Albrektsson, T. Quintessence Publishing Co., Chicago, Ill.

2. Johansson, C. and Albrektsson, T.: Integration of screw implants in the rabbit: A one-year followup of removal torque of titanium implants. Int. J. Oral Max. Implants. 2:69-75, 1987.

CHAPTER 3

Edentulous Bone Anchored Fixed Bridge

INTRODUCTION

The "Branemark" osseointegrated implant system was originally designed and utilized for the treatment of the edentulous mandible. The fixed bone-anchored bridge, anchored to four to six implant fixtures, was the most common restoration employed. This chapter will review the methods used to determine patient selection, prepare the investing soft tissues following abutment connection, detail the prosthetic procedures, and discuss oral hygiene and followup procedures.

DIAGNOSTIC PROCEDURES

The edentulous mandible often presents a difficult prosthetic challenge. Placement of osseointegrated implants and fabrication of an implant-supported fixed partial denture can greatly improve mastication and with it, the quality of life. The clinical exam should note the presence of soft tissue pathology or mucogingival abnormalities which may preclude the use of osseointegrated implants. The amount of keratinized attached mucosa is an important prognostic factor. Patients with insufficient attached mucosa may require grafting.

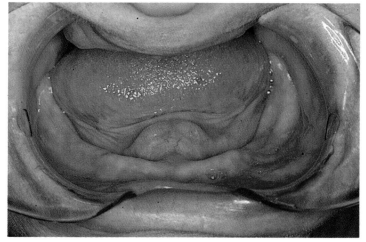

Fig. 3-1

RADIOGRAPHS

A panoramic radiograph is necessary in the evaluation of both bone quantity and quality. The number of fixtures required to support the definitive prosthesis is determined by the bone height (which dictates fixture length), bone quality, and the distance between the two mental foramen. The density of the trabecular pattern and the thickness of the cortical plates are key factors in predicting the quality of osseointegration.

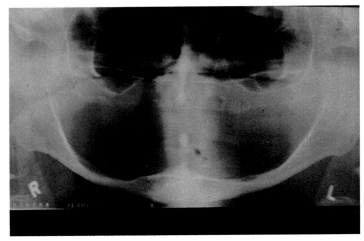

Fig. 3-2

Edentulous alveolar ridges may show various resorption patterns. Anatomic contours of the anterior ridge can be evaluated with the use of a lateral cephalometric radiograph. This is very helpful during the surgical placement of the implant fixtures. The thickness of cortical bone also can be seen easily.

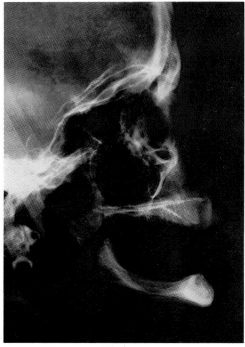

Fig. 3-3

DIAGNOSTIC CASTS

Ridge relationships will often dictate the design of the definitive prosthesis. Osseointegration does allow the restorative dentist some flexibility in tooth placement due to the ability to cantilever, but ridge anatomy may limit fixture placement. Mounted diagnostic casts are necessary to evaluate the probable tooth placement. A class I ridge relationship reduces potential difficulty, since both maxillary and mandibular anterior teeth will most likely be set somewhat to the labial of the resorbed ridges.

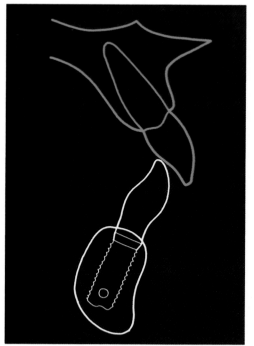

Fig. 3-4

A class II relationship may require substantial labial placement of mandibular anterior teeth. Implant fixtures placed with a slight labial inclination will reduce the labial-lingual dimension of the anterior portion of the bridge, allowing for easier cleansibility. Tongue function and speech may be compromised by a prosthesis with an excessive labial-lingual dimension.

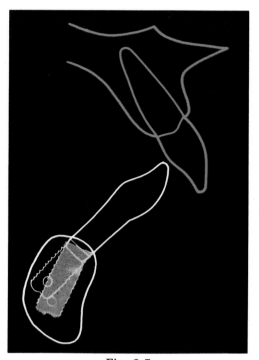

Fig. 3-5

Class III relationships often require slight lingual placement of the mandibular anterior teeth for patient satisfaction. Implants with a labial inclination would most probably create an esthetic problem due to the screw access holes being located on the labial surface of the teeth.

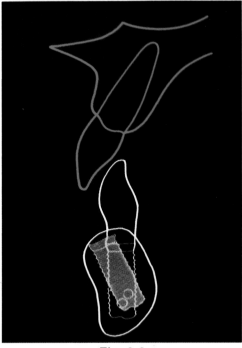

Fig. 3-6

SURGICAL PROCEDURES

Surgical Stents

In most cases, it is helpful to have presurgical knowledge of the approximate desired tooth position. Existing dentures may be duplicated in clear acrylic resin if no major changes are to be made. Otherwise, wax trial dentures with proper esthetics and function are fabricated, and then duplicated in clear acrylic resin. (Figs. 3-7,A and B.)

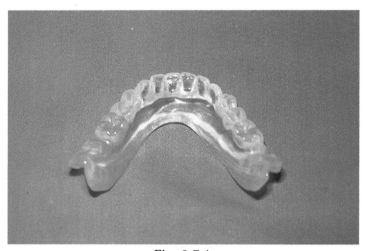

Fig. 3-7,A

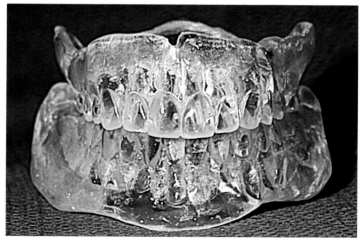

Fig. 3-7,B

The clear acrylic resin stents (Figs. 3-8, A and B) are trimmed so that they can be used as guides for fixture placement during surgery. The surgical incision will be made in the buccal vestibule and the tissue will be reflected lingually or palatally. The stent must not interfere with the reflected tissue; and the lingual aspects of the mandibular stent or palatal aspect of the maxillary must be removed.

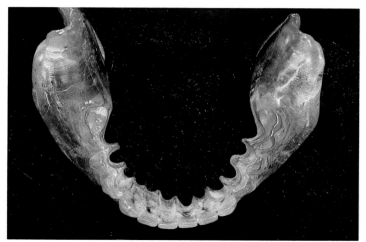

Fig. 3-8,A

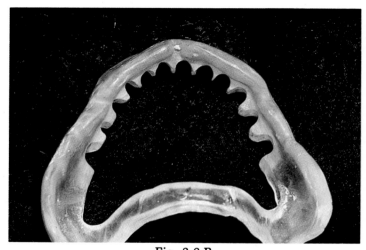

Fig. 3-8,B

Fixture Placement

It is important to reflect a large enough tissue flap to allow for good visibility and access during implant placement, and to identify the important anatomic structures such as the mental nerve. It must be remembered that the inferior alveolar nerve may run anterior to the mental foramen before looping back and exiting the bone. Trauma to the nerve may lead to anesthesia, paresthsia, or dysethesia.

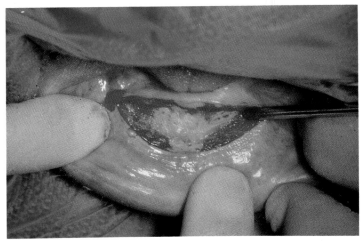

Fig. 3-9

With the aid of stents at the time of the implant installation, the surgeon will note the position of the teeth and should be able to place the fixtures in the proper location and in correct alignment so as to decrease the potential for future esthetic and functional compromises. (Figs. 3-10,A and B.)

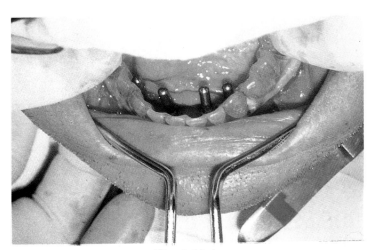

Fig. 3-10,A

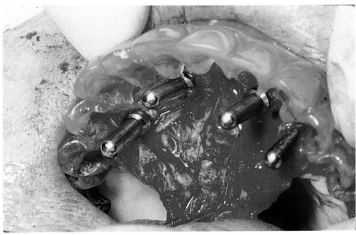

Fig. 3-10,B

The bone preparation prior to placement of the implant fixture is performed in a specific sequence utilizing various drills. It is critical to keep the temperature of the bone well below 47° centigrade in order to achieve effective bone healing and osseointegration. Higher temperatures may lead to bone necrosis and eventual fibrous connective tissue encapsulation of the implant fixture. Constant irrigation, as well as maintaining low handpiece speed, will allow for proper bone preparation and healing. While the implant system allows for significant angulation between fixtures, it is best to obtain parallelism as much as possible. Direction indicators can be placed in prepared bone sites and utilized as references during the surgical procedure.

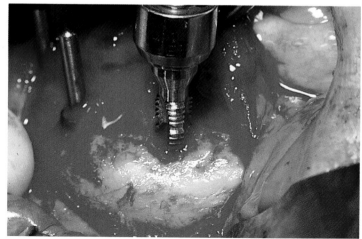

Fig. 3-11

The surgical system will tap the bone sites to a diameter of 3.5 mm. Irrigation, and a drill speed of no more than 15-20 RPMs, must be maintained at all times.

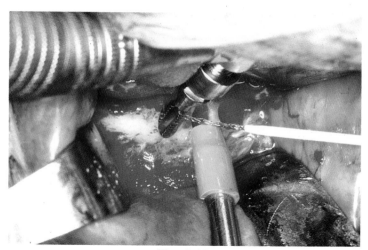

Fig. 3-12

Threads of the tapped bone site can be seen in this patient.

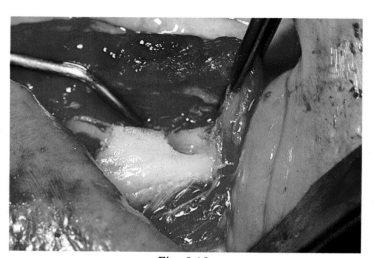

Fig. 3-13

The implant fixtures, which are 3.75 mm in diameter, are placed into the previously tapped surgical sites. Being slightly larger than the tapped bone diameter they will expand the bone and provide an extremely close adaptation between the titanium fixture and surrounding bone. Implant fixtures of 4.0 mm diameter are available should the implant site be stripped or over expanded. (Figs. 3-14,A and B.)

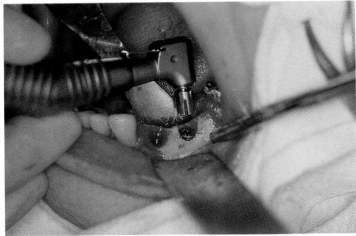

Fig. 3-14,A

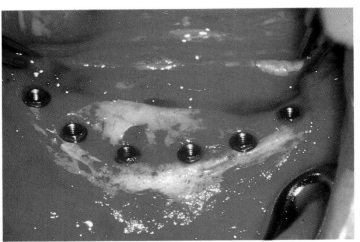

Fig. 3-14,B

The final tightening of the fixture into bone is performed with a hand wrench. The increased tactile sensation provided by this technique allows for greater precision in the final seating of the implant fixture. A titanium cover screw is then placed in order to maintain the opening for the abutment screw. (Figs. 3-15,A and B.)

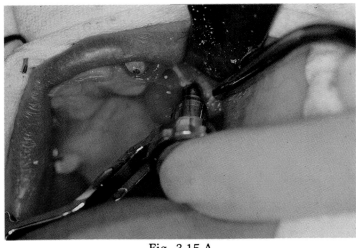

Fig. 3-15,A

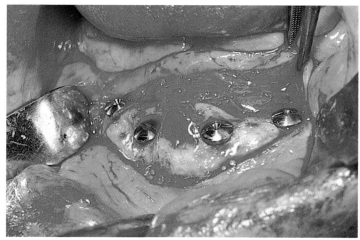

Fig. 3-15,B

The mucosal flaps are repositioned and securely sutured. Placement of the incision line in the labial/buccal vestibule rather than over the crest of the ridge is advised. This design helps to prevent exposure of the recently placed implant fixtures should a dehisence of the incision occur. It is also important that the patient not wear an existing prosthesis for the initial 10-14 day healing period. Trauma to the incision should be avoided to prevent tissue breakdown. Loading over the recently placed fixtures may cause loosening, and result in fibrous tissue encapsulation of the implant fixture.

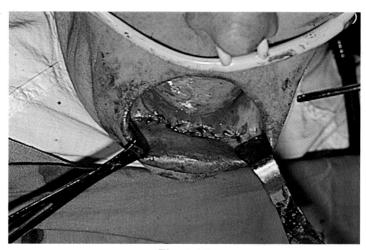

Fig. 3-16

POST SURGICAL TREATMENT

Following the 10-14 day initial healing period, the patient is ready for adaptation of their existing prosthesis. The sutures have been removed or have resorbed by this time. The soft tissues are evaluated to assure adequate healing. If exposure of an implant fixture and cover screw is noted, a surgical procedure may be necessary to close the tissues. Adaptation and placement of the prosthesis must then be delayed.

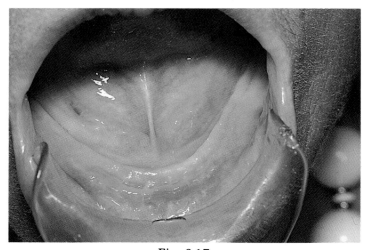

Fig. 3-17

Denture Alteration

The labial/buccal flange of the existing denture is generously relieved in order to prevent pressure or tension over the healing incision. The relief must extend distally beyond the distal-most fixture.

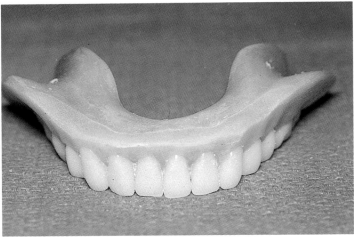

Fig. 3-18

Soft Tissue Conditioner

Tissue conditioning material is applied to the denture to provide a closely adapted cushion over the mucosa. Careful inspection is necessary to determine whether or not adequate buccal flange relief has been achieved. It may be necessary to remount and equilibrate the dentures to eliminate occlusal discrepancies.

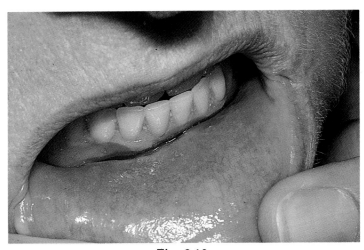

Fig. 3-19

A periodontal probe can be used to evaluate the thickness of the tissue-conditioning material. This is necessary to ensure adequate relief over the implant tissues; a thin layer of tissue conditioner may require further relief of the denture. During the next few weeks, several adjustments may be necessary to attain patient comfort. Following this period, the material should be changed as necessary.

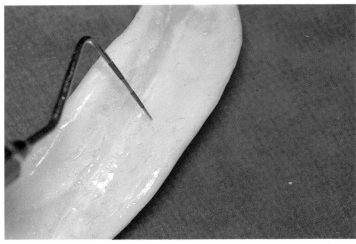

Fig. 3-20

A healing period of four months in the mandible is recommended prior to uncovering the implant fixtures and utilizing them prosthodontically. The maxilla, with a somewhat less dense cancellous bone, requires six to eight months to achieve a state of osseointegration. Unusually poor quality bone, as well as other factors such as placement of fixtures that are shorter than desired due to anatomic restrictions, are important in determining whether a lengthier healing time is advisable. It must be remembered that the quality of osseointegration continues to improve after the initial four to six month healing period, and is especially noticeable up to the first year.

ABUTMENT CONNECTION

During the second surgical procedure, the implant fixture is exposed, the cover screw removed, and the titanium abutment cylinder which emerges through the gingival tissues is attached. There are two different approaches to this procedure. Most surgeons prefer a long incision similar to the initial one, exposing all the fixtures with one flap. Others prefer smaller individual incisions over each fixture. The smaller "punch" type of incision can be utilized in situations where the fixtures are far apart and where there is ample attached keratinized tissue. When a submucosal resection is necessary, the long incision is employed.

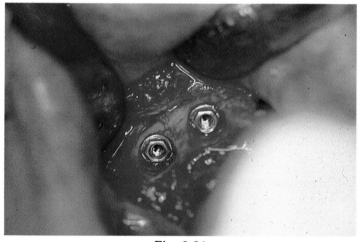

Fig. 3-21

In some instances, bone may have grown over the implant fixture and cover screw. Any new bone which may interfere with proper seating of the abutment must be removed.

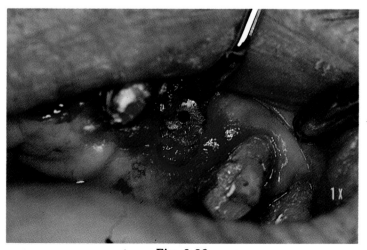

Fig. 3-22

The abutment is a titanium cylinder which fits directly on top of the implant fixture. The abutments come in various lengths, from 3 to 10 mm. Matching abutment screws are used to hold the abutments in place. The surgeon must decide which length is necessary to emerge through the gingival tissues. While the edentulous implant-supported fixed restoration should be 4-6 mm above the gingival crest, an implant-supported tissue bar utilized for an overdenture is usually closer to the soft tissues.

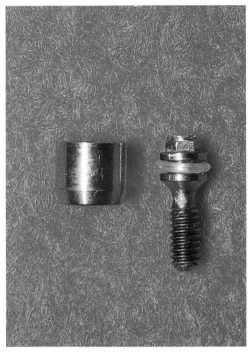

Fig. 3-23

The inferior aspect of the abutment cylinder has an internal hexagonal shape which matches the hexagon atop the implant fixture. This hexagon will prevent rotation of the abutment when secured to the fixture.

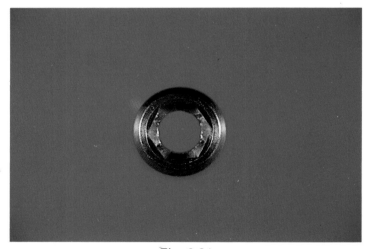

Fig. 3-24

The abutment cylinder cannot seat properly until the hexagons are lined up correctly. By rotating the abutment on top of the fixture, the abutment will slide into place in proper alignment.

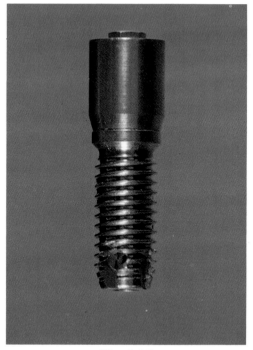

Fig. 3-25

A hemostat, designed to fit the contour of the abutment cylinder without scratching its surface, is used to secure the abutment cylinder in place while tightening the abutment screw.

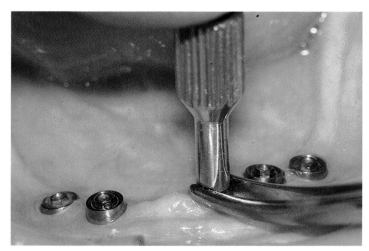

Fig. 3-26

To ensure proper seating of the abutment cylinder, a radiograph is taken to evaluate the abutment-fixture interface. Any noticeable gap is indicative of improper seating and the abutment should be removed. Entrapped tissue or debris must be removed if present, and the abutment connection repeated and confirmed with a new radiograph.

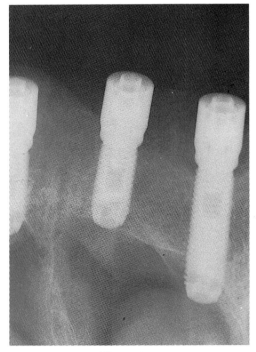

Fig. 3-27

This radiograph illustrates an abutment cylinder which is not completely seated into position.

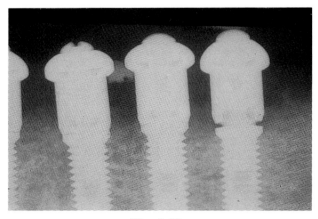

Fig. 3-28

Healing Caps

Plastic healing caps can be screwed into the internal aspect of the abutment screw. The hexagonal abutment screw driver fits the hexagonal pattern on top of the healing cap and can be used for placing and removing this component.

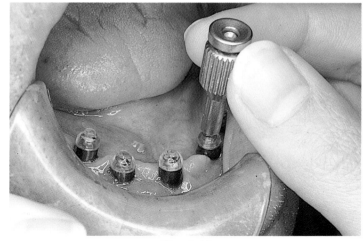

Fig. 3-29

In many instances the soft tissue, recently traumatized by the second surgical procedure, may become edematous and hypertrophic and extend above the abutment cylinder (Fig. 3-30,A). Impingement of the soft tissues between the denture and abutment can cause considerable patient discomfort.

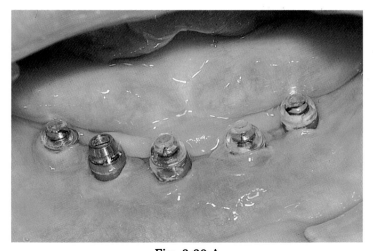

Fig. 3-30,A

The healing cap is placed and temporarily extends the abutment cylinder above the inflammed tissues, supporting the tissue during the healing process and facilitating oral hygiene (Fig. 3-30,B).

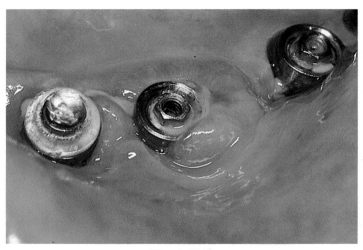

Fig. 3-30,B

After healing, if the abutment cylinder remains below the gingival crest, it should be replaced with a new longer abutment (Fig. 3-30,C).

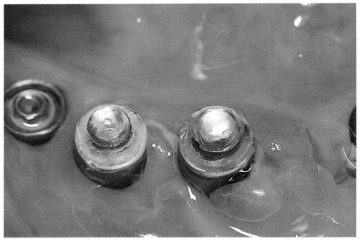

Fig. 3-30,C

After a short period of time (10-14 days) with the healing caps in place, soft tissue healing should occur. Initial hygiene in this sensitive area may be difficult to achieve. Hygiene is facilitated with the use of anti-plaque substances such as chlorhexidine gluconate.

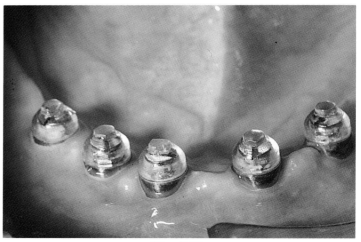

Fig. 3-31

Soft Tissue Management

Hygiene aids such as end tuft brushes will facilitate oral hygiene. Good oral hygiene practices must be stressed and developed at this early stage of treatment.

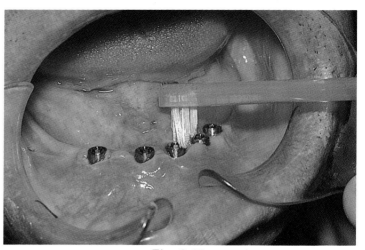

Fig. 3-32

The soft tissue response may be quite good just one or two weeks after the abutment connection, but it is most notable when an adequate amount of keratinized attached mucosa surrounds the abutment.

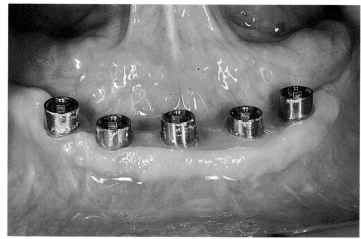

Fig. 3-33

Slow healing is often noted when the abutment cylinder is surrounded by a poorly keratinized non-attached mucosa. When combined with poor oral hygiene, edema and granulation tissue formation is even more pronounced.

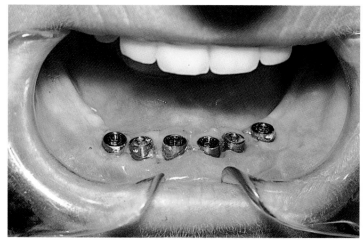

Fig. 3-34

Soft tissue hypertrophy is sometimes seen around one fixture while the others appear to have a quite good response. Meticulous hygiene and twice daily applications of chlorhexidine gluconate will promote healing.

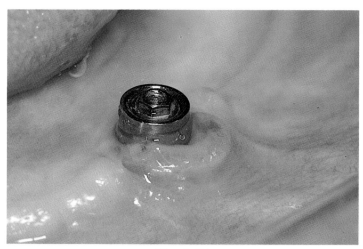

Fig. 3-35

When the abutment cylinder is at or below the gingival margin, the soft tissue tends to prolilferate over the abutment cylinder. The hygiene around this sensitive tissue is difficut, and entrapment of the soft tissues between the abutment cylinder and denture promotes continued inflammation and edema.

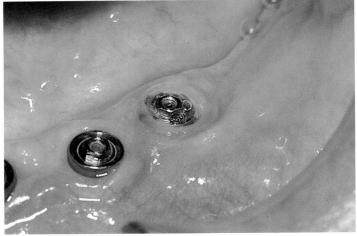

Fig. 3-36

By placing a healing cap, or in this case a gold cylinder, oral hygiene is facilitated and the tissue has a supportive matrix against which to heal.

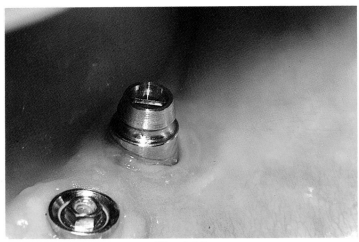

Fig. 3-37

The soft tissue healing is quite dramatic after just two or three days.

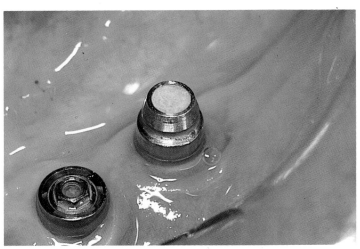

Fig. 3-38

Healing is complete within 7-10 days.

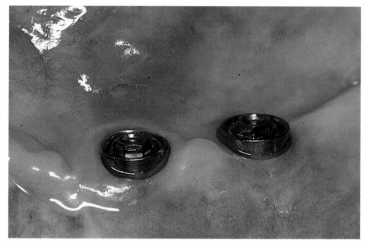

Fig. 3-39

When abutment cylinders are placed in mobile non-attached tissues, the tissue may proliferate, encompassing even the longest abutment.

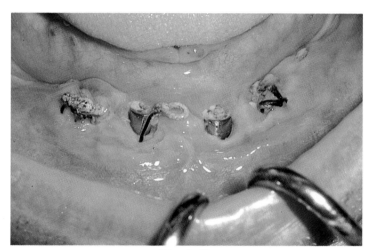

Fig. 3-40

In these extreme cases, neither healing caps nor gold cylinders may extend above the soft tissues. It may be necessary to place cylindrical impression copings to promote initial healing.

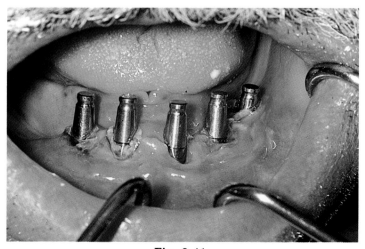

Fig. 3-41

Once initial soft tissue healing has occurred and the inflammation has subsided, the impression copings can be replaced with gold cylinders or healing caps.

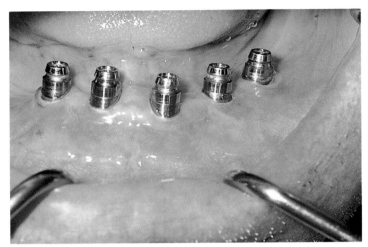

Fig. 3-42

Final healing is complete after a period of several weeks. This particular patient illustrates that dramatic soft tissue changes can occur without surgical intervention. Providing a smooth surface for the peri-implant tissue and maintaining good oral hygiene can result in significant tissue shrinkage and healing.

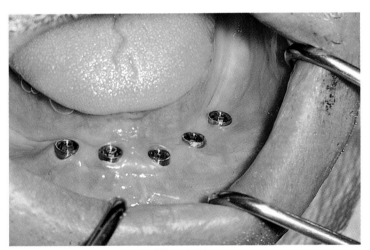

Fig. 3-43

A tissue graft may be necessary where excessive tissue mobility prevents adequate healing. Free palatal grafts are simple surgical procedures which provide an attached keratinized mucosal tissue around the abutment cylinder.

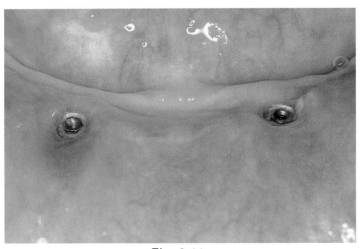

Fig. 3-44

A free palatal graft has been bucally to the crest of the ridge and is in the healing phase. This tissue will provide a more suitable environment around the abutment cylinders, allowing for improved hygiene.

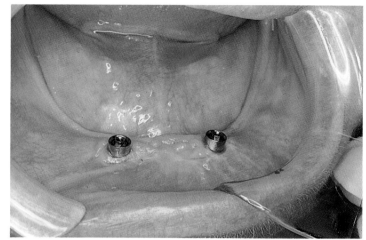

Fig. 3-45

Excessive tissue mobility on the lingual surface of the abutment cylinder presents a difficult situation. It is particularly important to avoid placement of the implant fixture in this highly mobile non-attached tissue bed.

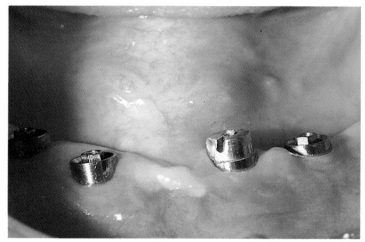

Fig. 3-46

A free palatal graft is sutured in place on the lingual surface of the abutment cylinder. Due to the high mobility of the lingual tissue, grafting is almost always necessary in these situations.

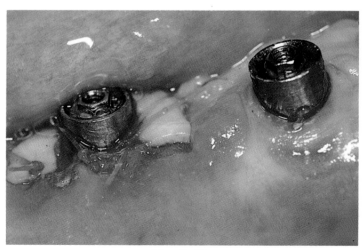

Fig. 3-47

Surgical stents can be attached to the abutments in order to hold the soft tissue grafts in place.

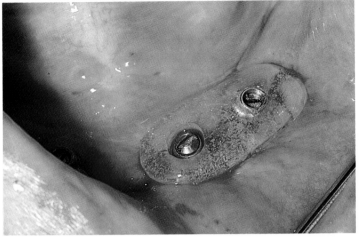

Fig. 3-48

Denture Adjustment

Once the abutment is positioned, the denture must be relieved so that it may be relined.

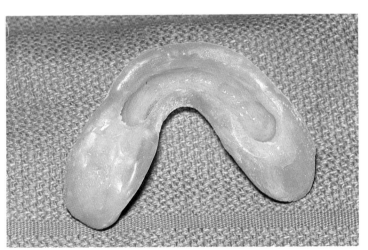

Fig. 3-49

Disclosing wax or pressure indicating paste can be placed in the relieved portion of the denture to determine if the relief is adequate (Fig. 3-50,A).

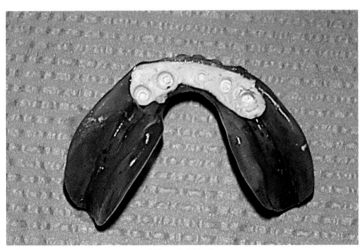

Fig. 3-50,A

An alternative method is to place the paste directly on the abutment cylinders and then seat the denture. The paste will transfer onto the inside of the denture where binding occurs (Fig. 3-50,B).

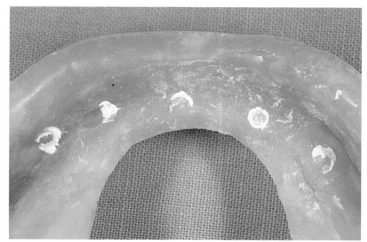

Fig. 3-50,B

Once relieved, the mandibular denture may be weak and susceptible to fracture. It is recommended to prevent fracture that acrylic resin be added to the lingual surface.

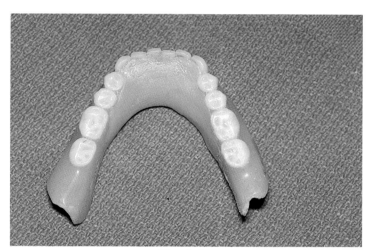

Fig. 3-51

A thick layer of tissue conditioner is placed inside, and the denture seated into position. This lining provides adequate adaptation and comfort, reduces irritation to the healing soft tissues, and prevents damage to abutment cylinders.

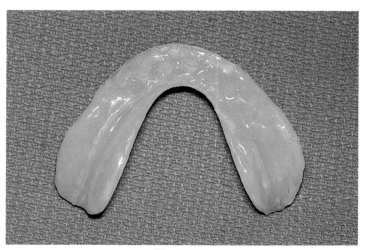

Fig. 3-52

The denture resin may contact the titanium abutments and loosen the abutment screws if there is insufficient relief of the denture over the abutment cylinders. It is important, therefore, that the abutment screws be checked for tightness prior to each restorative step.

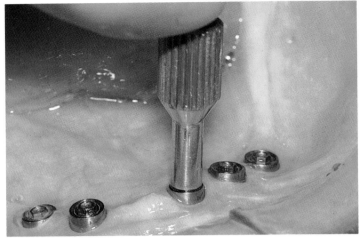

Fig. 3-53

Tissue hypertrophy encompassing an abutment may be an indication of a loose abutment screw and cylinder.

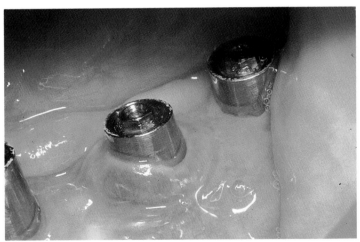

Fig. 3-54

The relatively soft titanium may be damaged if the removable prosthesis has metal components which come in contact with the abutment or abutment screw. It is important to remove any metal which may rest on or near the abutment to prevent this occurrence.

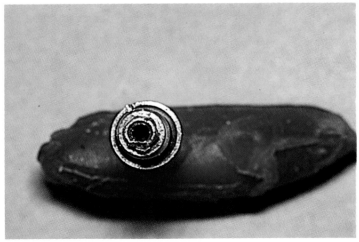

Fig. 3-55

Upon healing of the peri-implant tissues, the abutment cylinders should project 1½—2 mm above the tissue margins.

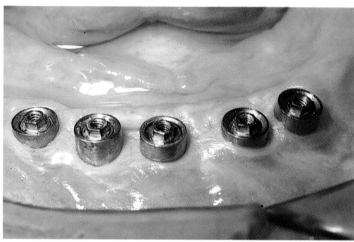

Fig. 3-56

PRELIMINARY IMPRESSIONS

Tapered Impression Copings

The tapered impression coping is designed to make preliminary impressions. This design allows the coping to remain screwed into the abutment when the impression is removed.

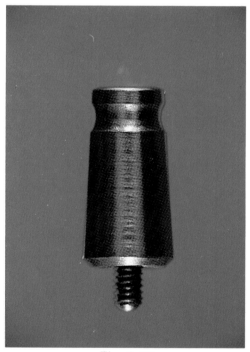

Fig. 3-57

A specially designed instrument grasps the impression coping and allows for easy insertion and removal of the coping.

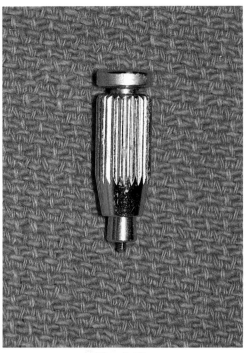

Fig. 3-58

The cylindrical copings should seat completely and firmly onto the abutments. The internal aspect of the abutment screws should be inspected and cleaned to ensure proper seating of the impression coping.

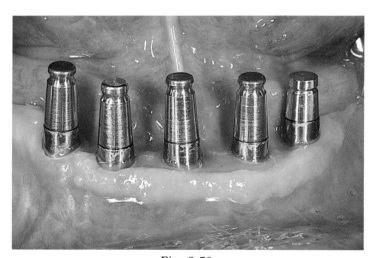

Fig. 3-59

A stock impression tray is utilized for the preliminary impression.

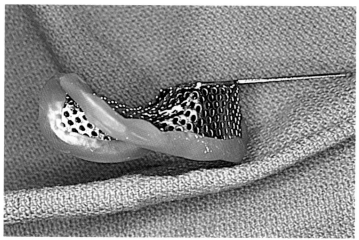

Fig. 3-60

The preliminary impression is made with irreversible hydrocolloid. The impression is removed, leaving the tapered impression copings attached to the abutments.

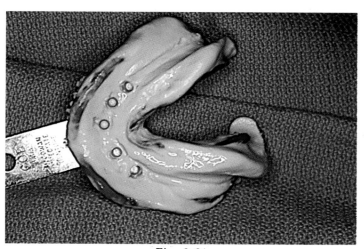

Fig. 3-61

Brass Analogues

This brass analogue will be used to represent the abutment cylinder during laboratory procedures.

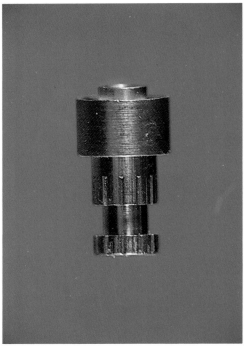

Fig. 3-62

The impression copings are removed from the mouth and connected to the brass analogues.

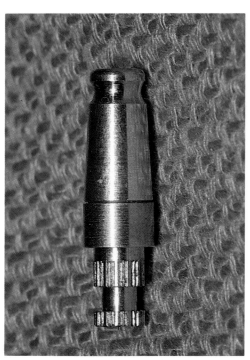

Fig. 3-63

Preliminary Cast

The impression copings are now inserted into the impression. It is important to seat the copings completely. The indented ring around the impression coping provides an undercut which will allow the coping to snap into proper position. The impression is poured with improved dental stone, taking care not to vibrate the copings out of position.

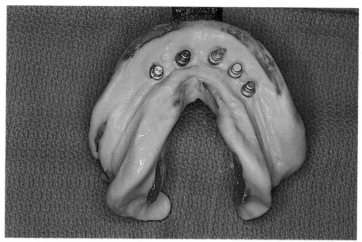

Fig. 3-64

The impression tray is removed, leaving the preliminary cast with the tapered impression copings in place and the brass analogues incorporated into the stone. The copings are removed, and fabrication of the master impression tray can begin.

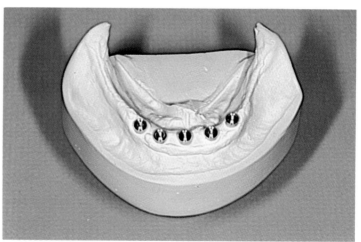

Fig. 3-65

MASTER IMPRESSIONS

Square Impression Copings

The square impression copings are used for master impressions. Their design allows them to become locked into the impression material. The impression cannot be removed from the oral cavity unless the guide screw, which connects the impression coping to the abutment, is loosened from the abutment screw.

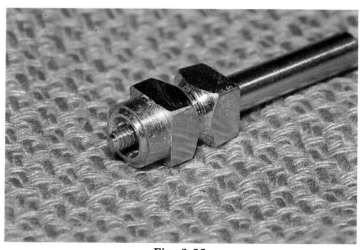

Fig. 3-66

This sectional view shows the impression coping locked into the impression material. Since it is not removed and repositioned into the impression, a source of error is eliminated.

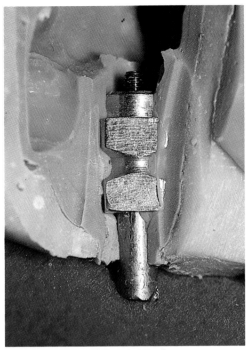

Fig. 3-67

The square impression copings are positioned on the preliminary cast and secured in place by the long guide screws (Figs. 3-68, A and B).

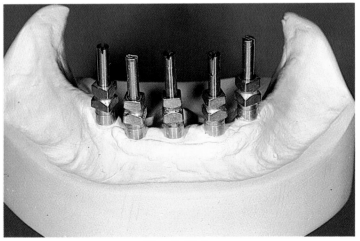

Fig. 3-68,A

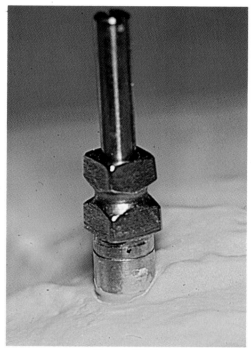

Fig. 3-68,B

If adjustments to the square copings are necessary to enable proper positioning, it should be accomplished during this step rather than at chairside.

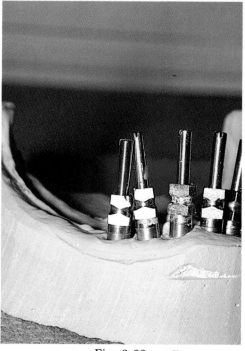

Fig. 3-69

Custom Tray Fabrication

Wax relief around the impression copings is provided prior to fabrication of the master impression tray. This will allow a sufficient thickness of impression material around the impression copings.

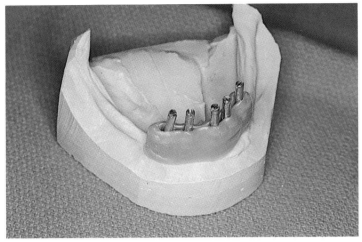

Fig. 3-70

The master impression tray is fabricated with tray resin. The long guide screws must be accessible, since the impression cannot be removed intraorally until they are loosened. It is also important that the impression tray cover the retromolar pads, since they are important landmarks in determining the occlusal plane of the final restoration.

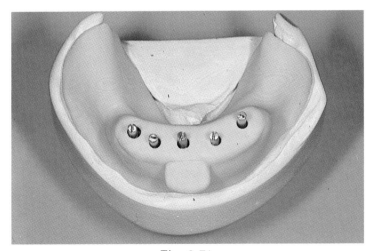

Fig. 3-71

The undersurface of the tray is smoothed to prevent irritation to the soft tissues.

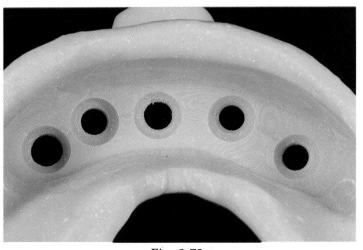

Fig. 3-72

Impression Techniques

The abutment cylinders are cleaned and tightened prior to placement of the impression copings. If either the abutment cylinders or copings are not secured firmly in place, the impression will be inaccurate. It is important that necessary changes in abutment heights be made prior to making the final impression.

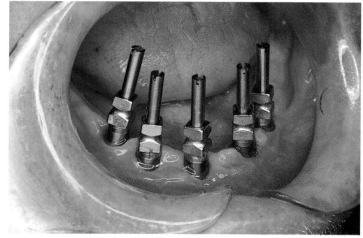

Fig. 3-73

The impression tray is positioned over the impression copings. If the long guide screws or impression copings interfere with the placement of the impression tray, the tray must be relieved. Once adjusted, the inner surface of the tray is painted with impression adhesive.

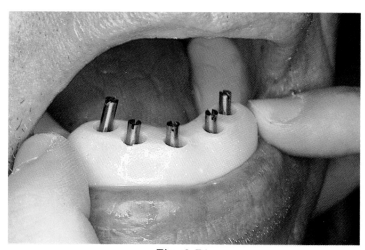

Fig. 3-74

There are several impression materials and methods in use at present. Some recommend creating a rigid matrix to relate and hold the impression copings together. With this technique, floss is tied around the copings to provide a scaffolding for the material of choice.

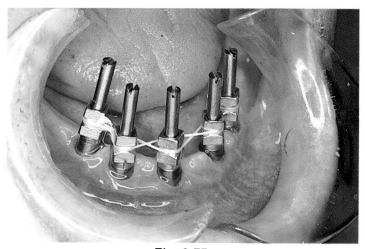

Fig. 3-75

Duralay[1] is used as a matrix in this case. Once polymerized, the Duralay[1] acts to hold the copings together in proper relationship to each other within the master impression.

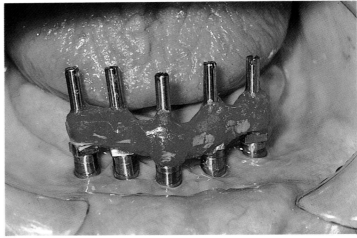

Fig. 3-76

The impression must accurately reflect the positions of the abutment cylinders. Osseointegrated implants exhibit no mobility; there is little room for error. Consequently, the contracture associated with a large bulk of acrylic resin may result in an inaccurate relationship. Alternate methods have been developed which diminish or eliminate the effects of polymerization on the accuracy of the impression. In this case, acrylic resin was added to the square impression copings on the preliminary cast (Fig. 3-77,A).

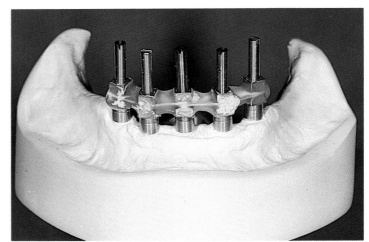

Fig. 3-77,A

The resin is then sectioned with a thin separating disc (Fig. 3-77,B).

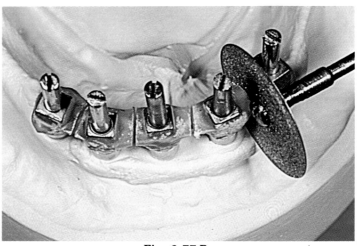

Fig. 3-77,B

The impression copings with resin are placed intraorally and then luted together. This technique results in minimal distortion.

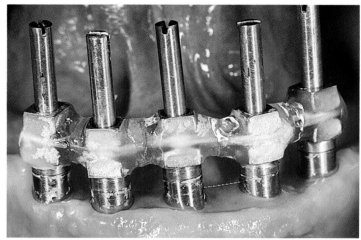

Fig. 3-78

Experience has shown that in most cases no supportive matrix is necessary. Medium or heavy body polyvinyl siloxanes or polyether impression materials will result in an accurate impression, with or without supportive matrices.

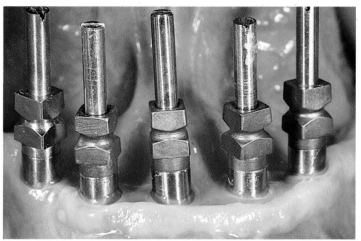

Fig. 3-79

Once the impression material is syringed around the copings and/or supportive matrix, the tray is filled with heavy bodied material and positioned. It is useful to remove excess material around the guide screws before the material polymerizes.

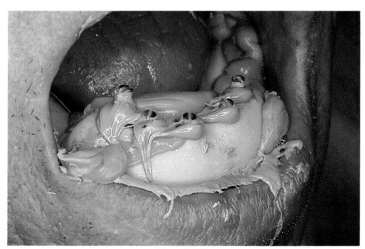

Fig. 3-80

The square impression copings must be released from the abutments to remove the impression tray from the mouth. The guide screws are loosened completely to accomplish this task. Once they are disengaged from the abutments, the tray is removed. The guide screws should be left in the impression, since they will be needed to attach the brass analogues. Removing and then reinserting the guide screws could distort the impression.

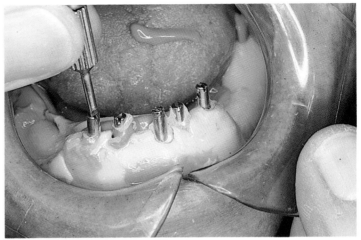

Fig. 3-81

The master impression displays the bottom of the impression copings. Also noteworthy is the presence of the retromolar pads.

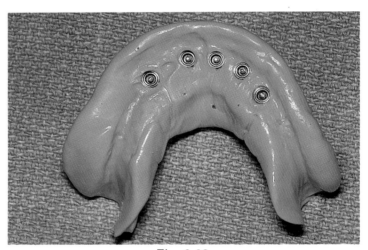

Fig. 3-82

Close inspection of the impression copings will reveal impression material which may have come between the impression copings and the abutments. If this occurs, a new impression is necessary. An acceptable impression is shown.

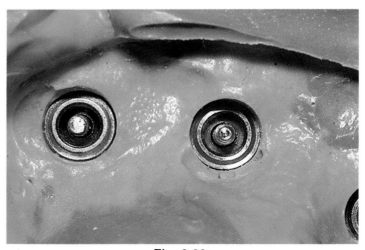

Fig. 3-83

The brass analogues are connected to the impression copings with the long guide screws (Figs. 3-84,A and B). Care must be taken to avoid rotation of the impression copings within the impression material when connecting the bass analogues.

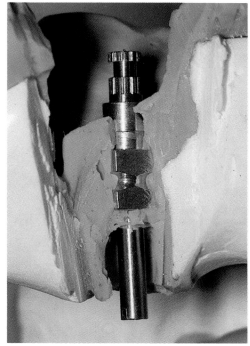

Fig. 3-84,A

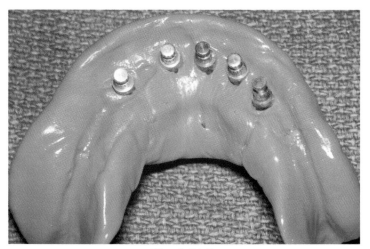

Fig. 3-84,B

The master impression is boxed and poured with an improved dental stone. The manufacturers' recommended water/powder ratios are strictly followed.

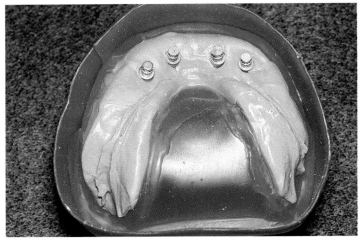

Fig. 3-85

Master Casts

The guide screws are disengaged and the impression tray removed revealing the master cast. If trimming of the cast is necessary, the retromolar pads and a significant land area must be retained. The final opposing cast should also be fabricated at this time.

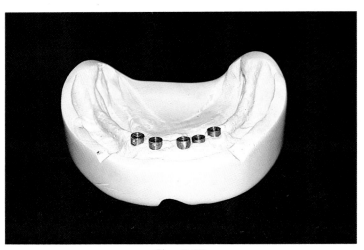

Fig. 3-86

INTEROCCLUSAL REGISTRATIONS

Gold-palladium Cylinders

Gold cylinders are available in both 3.0 mm and 4.0 mm heights, each with a corresponding gold screw. They engage onto the abutment cylinders as illustrated in this figure. These gold cylinders become incorporated into the final prosthesis, providing the means of attachment between the restoration and the abutments. At this stage they are utilized to fabricate the record base and trial denture.

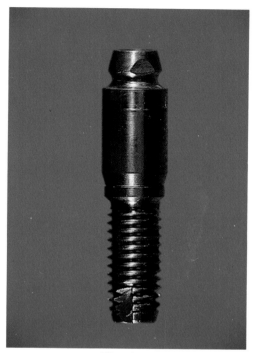

Fig. 3-87

The gold cylinders are positioned on the master cast and held in place with the laboratory guide screws. These gold cylinders will become incorporated into the record base.

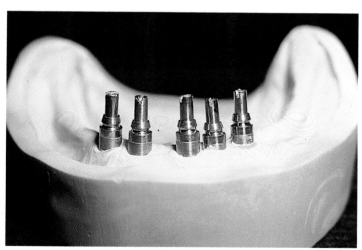

Fig. 3-88

Record Base

Prior to adding the acrylic resin, portions of the stone cast and gold cylinders are blocked out with wax. It is not necessary to totally envelope the gold cylinders with resin.

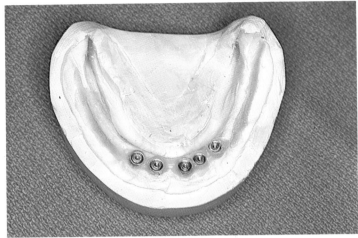

Fig. 3-89

Acrylic resin is applied to the cast to form the record base.

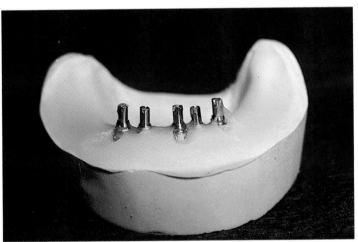

Fig. 3-90

The record base is trimmed and polished. The gold cylinders must be free of acrylic resin and debris to allow proper seating.

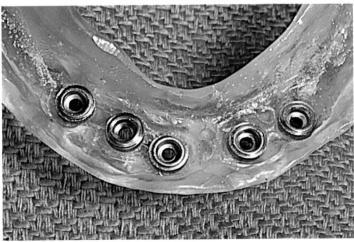

Fig. 3-91

The buccal aspect of the record base is removed. This allows visual inspection of the interface between the gold cylinders and abutment cylinders as the record base is seated intraorally.

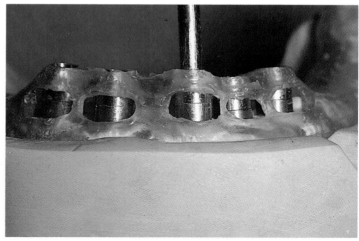

Fig. 3-92

The record base is trimmed and polished, and wax rims are added. The use of one or two short guide screws is necessary to adequately secure the record base in position intraorally. (Figs. 3-93,A and B.)

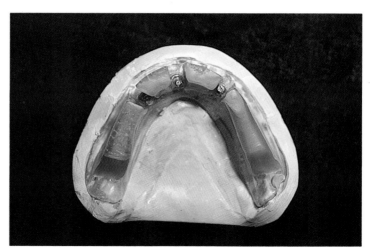

Fig. 3-93,A

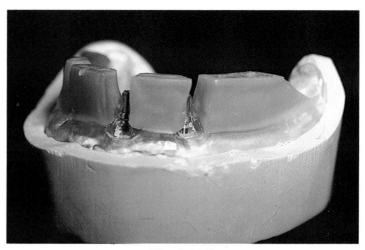

Fig. 3-93,B

Arbitrary Hinge Axis—Facebow Transfer

A facebow transfer record is made to position the maxillary cast on the articulator. (Figs. 3-94,A and B.)

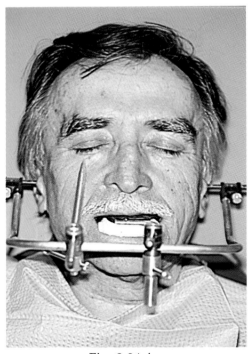

Fig. 3-94,A

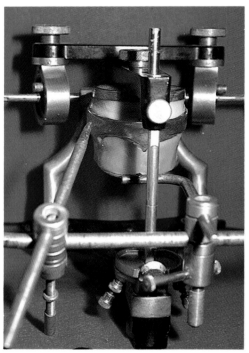

Fig. 3-94,B

Centric Relation

The centric relation record is made at the proper vertical dimension of occlusion. The mandibular record base, held securely in place by the short guide screws, enables the clinician to make accurate and reproducible records. Denture teeth are selected during this appointment.

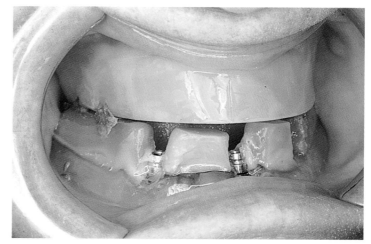

Fig. 3-95

The centric relation record is transferred to the articulator.

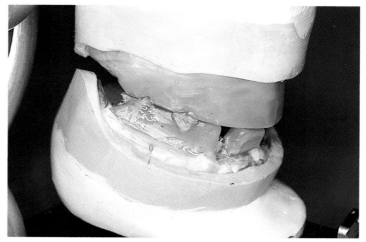

Fig. 3-96

TRIAL DENTURES

Cast Preparation

The prosthesis can extend no more than 20 mm distal to the center of the distal-most mandibular fixtures. The casts are marked to provide reference points during the positioning of denture teeth.

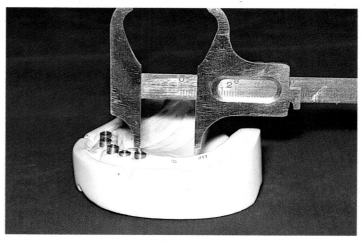

Fig. 3-97

The trial dentures are prepared in the usual fashion. The posterior occlusion is terminated short of the 20 mm mark in this patient.

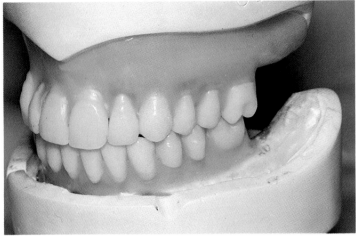

Fig. 3-98

Tooth Selection

Anatomic or nonanatomic teeth may be used for the edentulous fixed bone anchored bridge. It is recommended that plastic denture teeth be utilized rather than porcelain. In patients where the opposing prosthesis is a complete denture or an implant-supported overlay denture, bilaterally balanced occlusion is preferred. In patients presenting with severe maxillary atrophy, nonanatomic denture teeth are used. Unusual maxillo-mandibular relationships may also dictate the use of nonanatomic posterior denture teeth. When using nonanatomic teeth, a neutrocentric occlusal scheme is preferred.

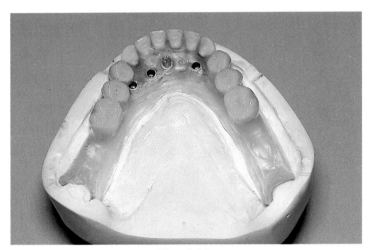

Fig. 3-99

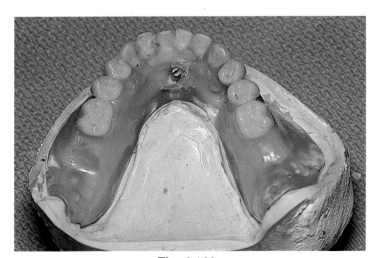

The trial denture is secured intraorally with one or two short guide screws.

Fig. 3-100

Utilizing all five gold cylinders does not require preparing screw access holes through several teeth. Since exact tooth position may not be determined at this stage, there is no point in drilling through a tooth which eventually may not be positioned over a gold cylinder.

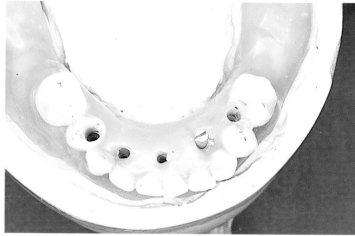

Fig. 3-101

Clinical Try-in

The vertical dimension of occlusion, centric relation, and esthetics are verified at the clinical try-in appointment.

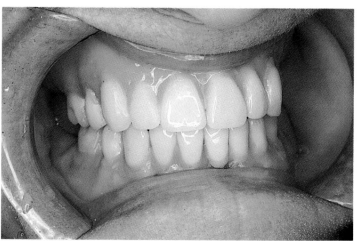

Fig. 3-102

Protrusive Records

Modeling plastic was used in this patient to make the protrusive record.

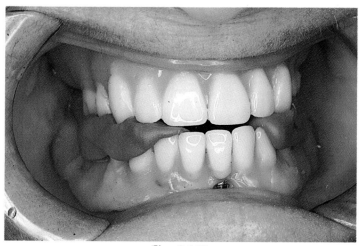

Fig. 3-103

The condylar inclinations are set according to the protrusive record.

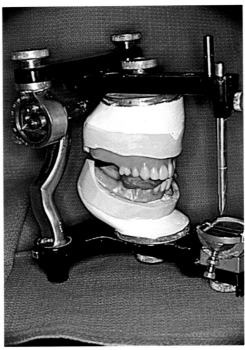

Fig. 3-104

METAL FRAMEWORK FABRICATION

With the trial denture complete, the metal substructure for the definitive prosthesis is fabricated. It is important that framework contours be compatible with the position of the teeth. For this reason it is necessary to record the position of the teeth in a matrix and use this matrix as a guide during fabrication of the framework. Either silicone or stone can be used. Stone is preferred because it provides a more stable matrix and retains the teeth more effectively. The matrix material should encompass the buccal and occlusal surfaces of the trial denture, and can be repositioned by engaging the notches in the land of the cast.

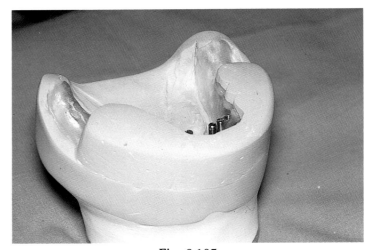

Fig. 3-105

The lingual surfaces of the teeth and trial denture are not covered by the matrix.

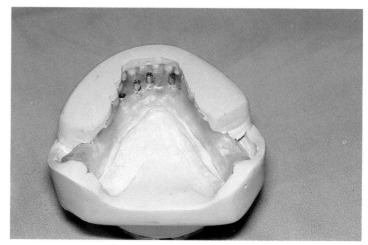

Fig. 3-106

The matrix is removed from the trial denture. The teeth are removed and placed in the matrix. They are held in position with a small drop of wax.

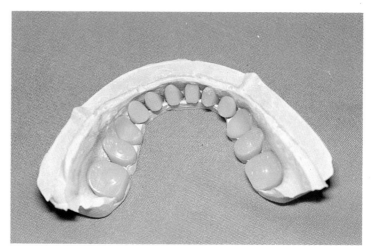

Fig. 3-107

The record base and wax are discarded. Gold cylinders, which will become incorporated in the final framework, are positioned onto the cast. If possible, laboratory guide screws are used rather than the gold screws.

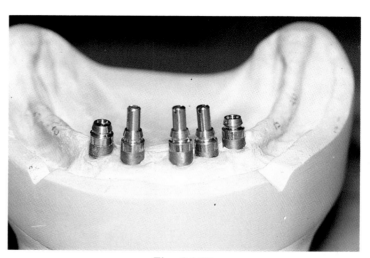

Fig. 3-108

The matrix, with the teeth in place, is positioned on the cast. This provides the laboratory technician a perspective of the space available for the framework.

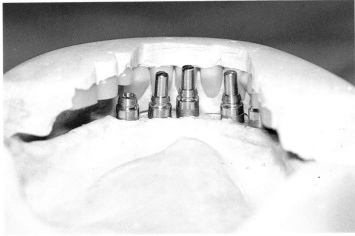

Fig. 3-109

This close-up view shows the relationship between the gold cylinders and the denture teeth.

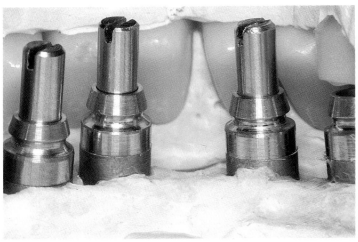

Fig. 3-110

Wax Pattern

Fabrication of the framework begins by placing plastic bars between the gold cylinders. The matrix is frequently positioned to insure correct development of the framework pattern.

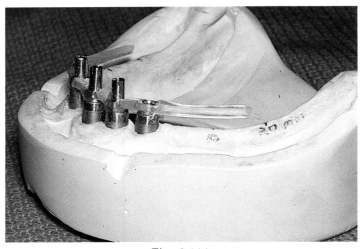

Fig. 3-111

Wax is added to continue framework fabrication.

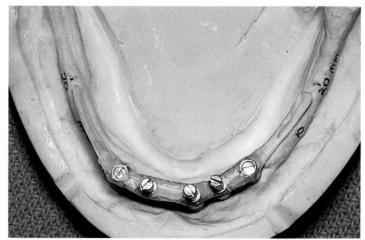

Fig. 3-112

The wax pattern is reinforced in selected areas to avoid fracture of the finished restoration. The most critical areas are adjacent to the distal-most implant fixtures.

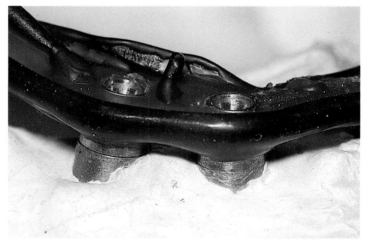

Fig. 3-113

Beads and loops are added to the wax pattern for purposes of acrylic resin retention.

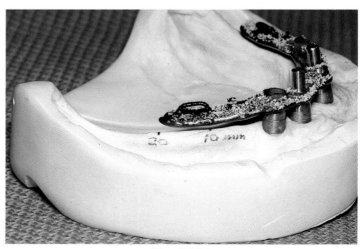

Fig. 3-114

It is best to place the teeth and framework over the ridge or slightly to the buccal. There is a degree of freedom in tooth placement with a bone anchored fixed bridge, since it is no longer necessary to place the teeth directly over the crest of the ridge. Positioning lingually may interfere with tongue space and may not provide sufficient facial support.

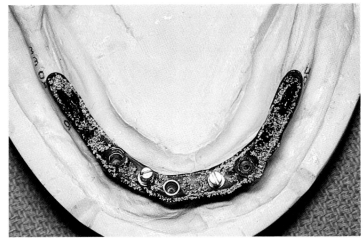

Fig. 3-115

The matrix is placed to insure that the completed wax pattern is compatible with the position of teeth.

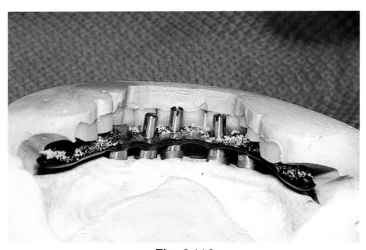

Fig. 3-116

This close-up lingual view shows the posterior matrix, teeth, and wax pattern.

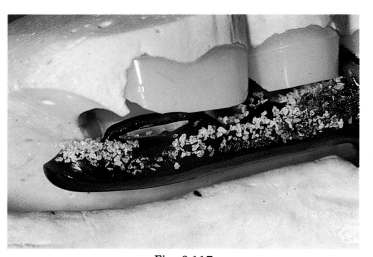

Fig. 3-117

The relationship of the anterior teeth and wax pattern is illustrated.

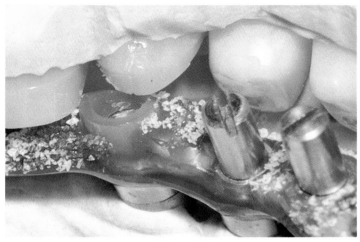

Fig. 3-118

The wax pattern should be terminated 2 mm short of the base of the gold cylinder. This prevents metal from flowing over the margin and into the inner aspect of the cylinder during castino. This practice enables easy finishing of the metal framework without damaging the gold cylinders, and allows access for oral hygiene.

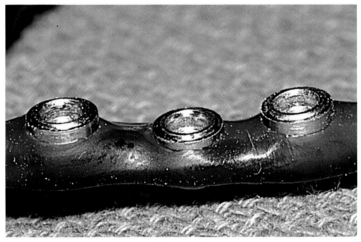

Fig. 3-119

It is important that a space of at least 4 mm exists between the soft tissues and the framework. A space of less than 4 mm would result in food impaction and impaired oral hygiene access.

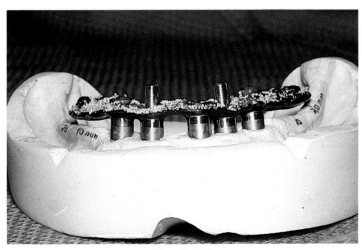

Fig. 3-120

The contour of the tissue surface of the framework must be convex to facilitate cleansibility. Concave surfaces become plaque traps and removal of the bridge would be necessary to maintain adequate hygiene.

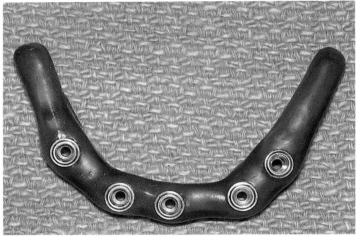

Fig. 3-121

The buccal-lingual dimension of the prosthesis must be kept minimal in order to facilitate access for oral hygiene. Too wide a surface will result in an uncleansible platform, allowing the accumulation of plaque and debris.

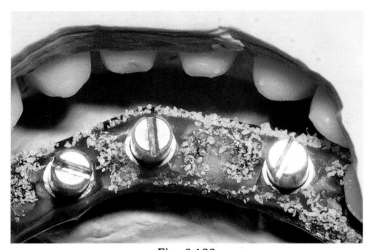

Fig. 3-122

The wax pattern may incorporate various stresses during its fabrication. Removal of the wax pattern from the cast may allow these stresses to distort the pattern, resulting in an inaccurate casting. In order to prevent this complication, the wax pattern can be sectioned between each implant fixture, allowing the stresses to dissipate. After a short period of time, the wax segments are luted together with cyanoacrylate, and the pattern is sprued and invested.

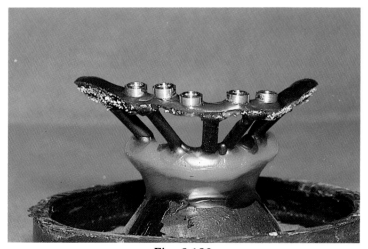

Fig. 3-123

Metal Casting

The completed silver-palladium casting is cleaned of investment material and is ready to be finished and polished.

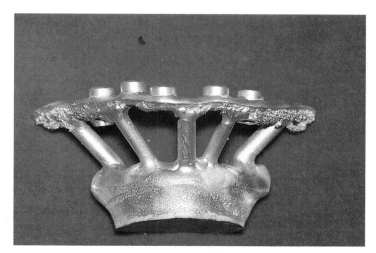

Fig. 3-124

Finishing and Polishing

Brass analogues can be used to protect the gold cylinders during finishing and polishing. Damage to the cylinders may prevent proper seating of the casting.

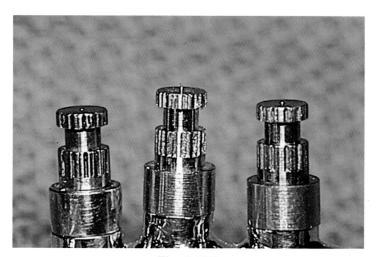

Fig. 3-125

The inner aspect of the gold cylinder should be visually inspected under a microscope to facilitate removal of excess metal and investment that may be present.

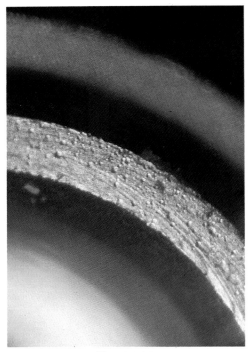

Fig. 3-126

The adaptation of the casting is verified on the master cast. In Figure 3-127,A the casting is well adapted to the brass analogues but the casting in Figure 3-127,B is poorly adapted.

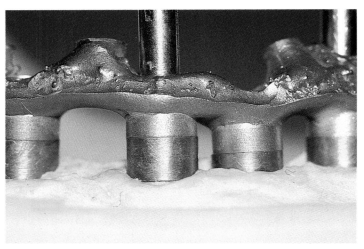

Fig. 3-127,A

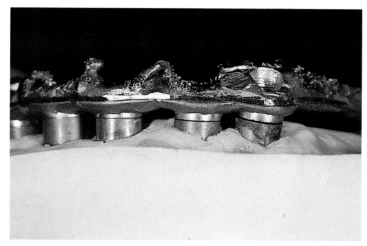

Fig. 3-127,B

The distal cantelever must maintain a constant 4-6 mm separation from the underlying soft tissues (Fig. 3-128,A).

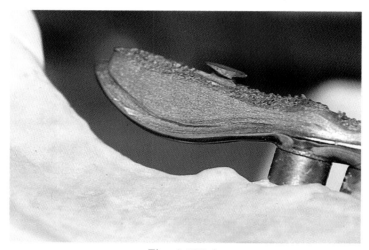

Fig. 3-128,A

Excessive space (Fig. 3-128,B) may lead to undesirable tongue manipulations.

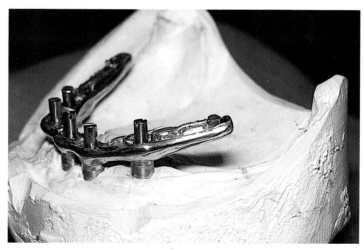

Fig. 3-128,B

Finishing and Polishing

When finishing and polishing the metal framework, brass analogues are connected to protect the exposed surfaces of the gold cylinders.

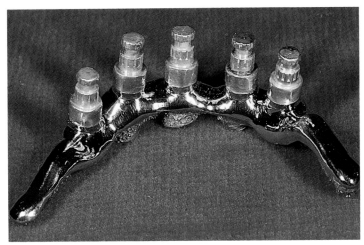

Fig. 3-129

FRAMEWORK TRY-IN

Clinical

The abutment cylinders are cleaned and tightened, and the framework is positioned. The design of the implant system allows for convergence or divergence of up to 40 degrees between fixtures. The framework should seat passively. The slightest discrepancy must be corrected.

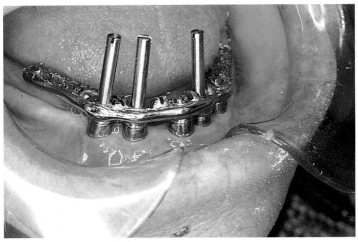

Fig. 3-130

Solder Relationship

If the framework exhibits a seating discrepancy, it is sectioned accordingly. Each segment must seat passively in position with no detectable movement or space between the gold cylinder and abutment.

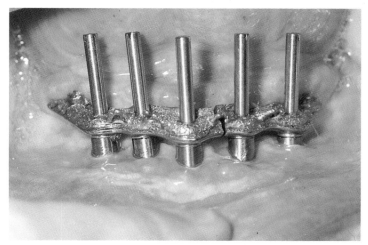

Fig. 3-131

With each section secured in place Duralay[1] is added to join the segments together.

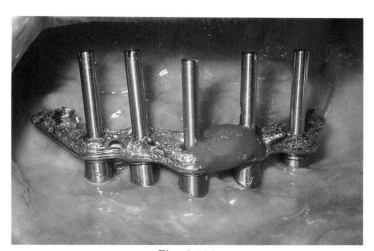

Fig. 3-132

The casting is then removed. Duralay[1] must be added to the exposed area of the solder joints. It is advantageous to place the framework back in the mouth to insure that no distortion has occurred.

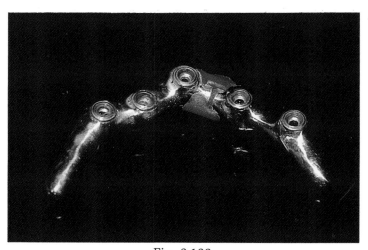

Fig. 3-133

Master Cast Alteration

In order to seat the altered framework onto the original model, one or more brass analogues must be repositioned. These analogues are removed and the stone model generously relieved in these areas.

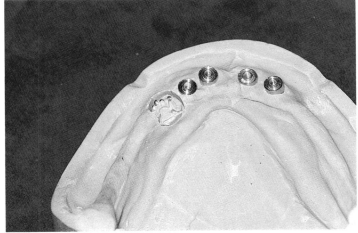

Fig. 3-134

With the analogues removed and connected to the framework, the framework is seated to insure that adequate stone has been removed around the newly positioned abutment analogues.

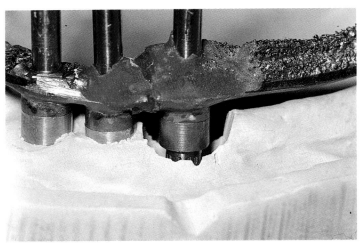

Fig. 3-135

Stone is added to the cast to secure the repositioned analogues in place. The framework is then removed and soldered.

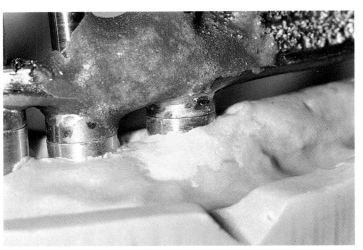

Fig. 3-136

The soldered framework is repositioned onto the altered model to verify solder joint accuracy. If distortions have occurred,they will be noted and a new solder record can be made, eliminating the need to recall the patient for another solder relation. The framework should be verified intraorally to ensure the accuracy of the original solder relationship.

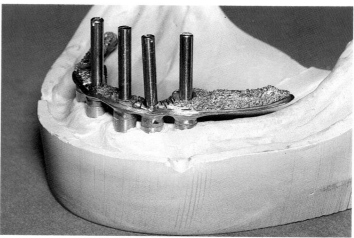

Fig. 3-137

PROCESSING

Repositioning Teeth

The verified casting is repositioned onto the master cast. The matrix and teeth are placed into position.

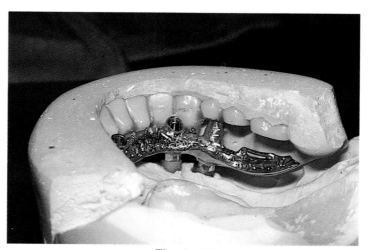

Fig. 3-138

Wax is added to join the teeth to the metal framework.

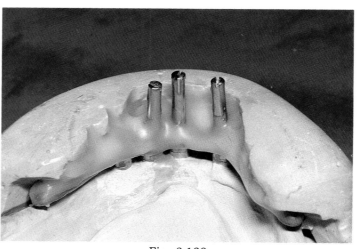

Fig. 3-139

Distortion of the wax often alters the positioning of the denture teeth. Occlusal contacts and wax contours must be re-established. (Figs. 3-140,A and B.)

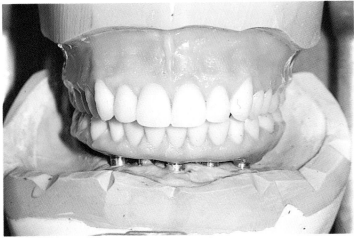

Fig. 3-140,A

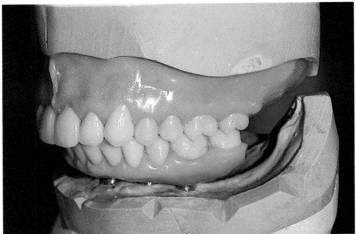

Fig. 3-140,B

During the final wax try-in appointment, the vertical dimension of occlusion and centric relation are verified. Minor esthetic changes also can be accomplished. Upon approval from the patient, the prosthesis is ready to be processed.

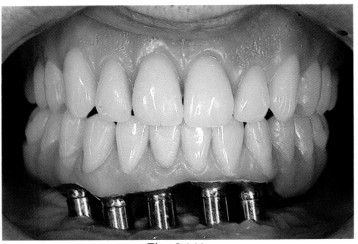

Fig. 3-141

Investing

In order to preserve the original model it is not used in flasking and investing. Holes are drilled through denture teeth as necessary to allow the connection of brass analogues to each gold cylinder, and the prosthesis and analogues are invested. (Figs. 3-142,A and B.)

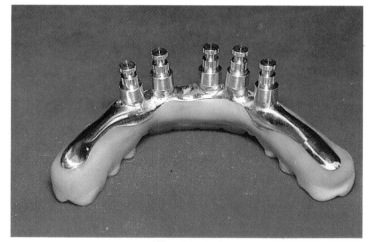

Fig. 3-142,A

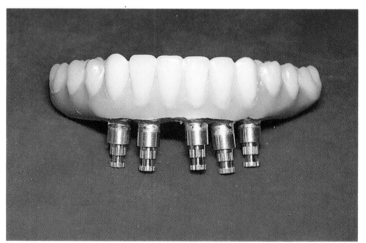

Fig. 3-142,B

Plaster is added to the brass analogues and undersurface of the bridge.

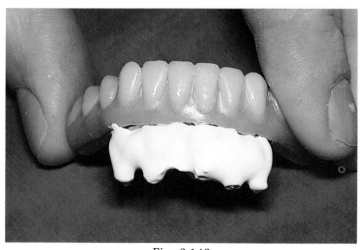

Fig. 3-143

The prosthesis is placed in the flask, submerging the brass analogues

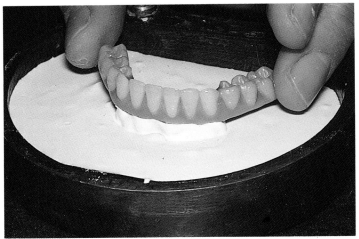

Fig. 3-144

The first layer of plaster is smoothed as shown.

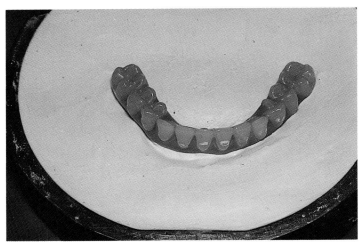

Fig. 3-145

A second layer of vacuum mixed stone is added to encompass the prosthesis. A third layer is then added to complete the investing process.

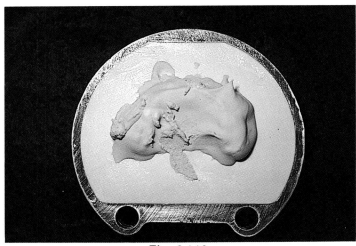

Fig. 3-146

Following wax elimination, the top half of the flask contains the denture teeth. Releasing agent is placed on the stone surfaces and diatorics are placed into the teeth to enhance acrylic retention.

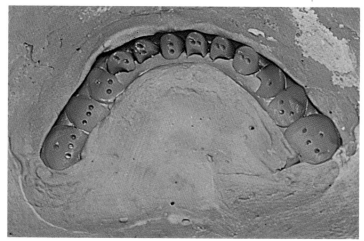

Fig. 3-147

The lower half of the flask contains the brass analogues, metal framework, and short guide screws.

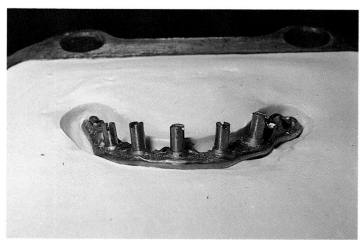

Fig. 3-148

Temporary cement is placed over the exposed guide screws. This facilitates removal of the guide screws following processing. Releasing agent is then placed over the plaster surface.

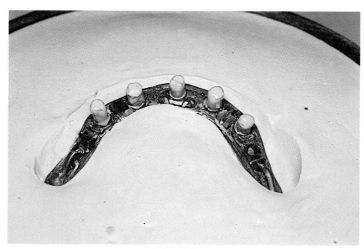

Fig. 3-149

Processing

The split-pack technique is used during trial packing.

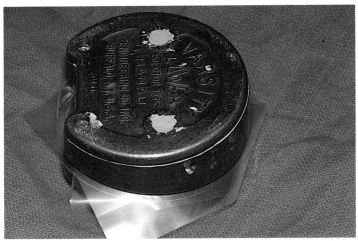

Fig. 3-150

After initial packing, the flask is opened. Acrylic resin is found in both halves.

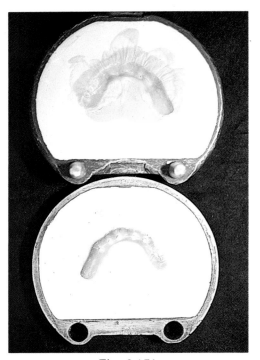

Fig. 3-151

Excess acrylic resin is trimmed in the usual fashion.

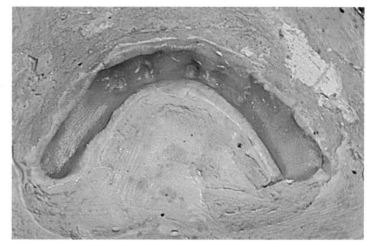

Fig. 3-152

The trial packing continues with increasing pressures until minimal flash results. The final packing is then performed and the acrylic resin is processed.

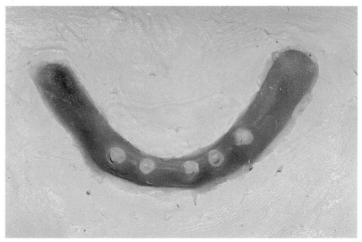

Fig. 3-153

Once processed, the flask is opened and the restoration removed.

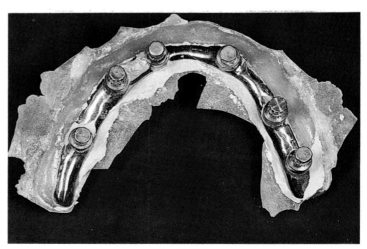

Fig. 3-154

Finishing

The excess acrylic resin and stone are removed, making sure to avoid damaging the gold cylinders.

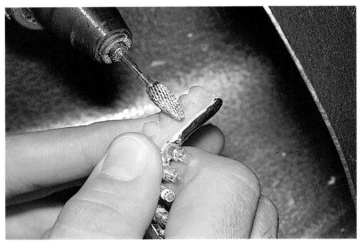

Fig. 3-155

The acrylic resin is finished and polished (Figs. 3-156, A and B) Note that the brass analogues are retained during polishing (Fig. 3-156,C).

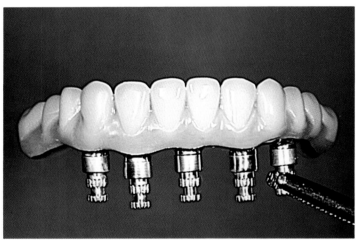

Fig. 3-156,A

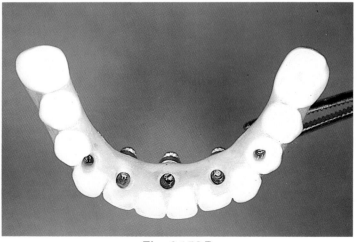

Fig. 3-156,B

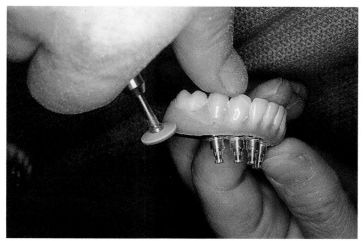

Fig. 3-156,C

A finished restoration is shown. Note the tapering contours designed to facilitate oral hygiene access.

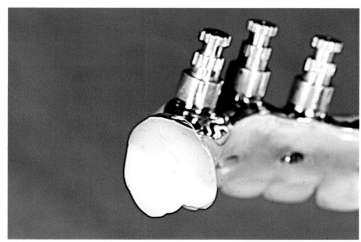

Fig. 3-157,A

Raising the metal-acrylic resin junction into a more accessible area decreases plaque accumulation.

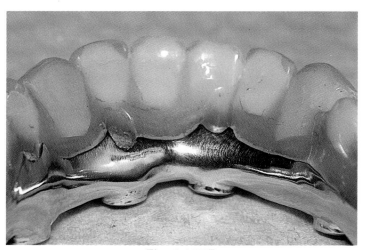

Fig. 3-157,B

DELIVERY

The restoration is secured with gold screws and a remount record retrieved (Figs. 3-158, A and B).

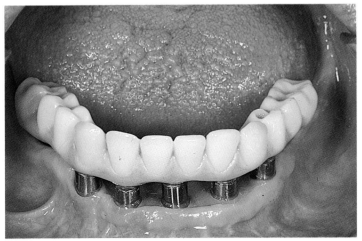

Fig. 3-158,A

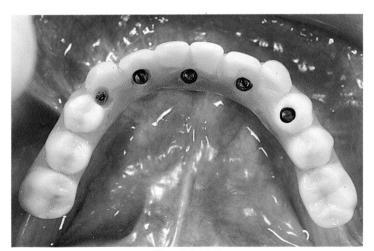

Fig. 3-158,B

Clinic Remount

New centric relation and protrusive records are made and the restoration is remounted. Posterior centric contacts should be confirmed and the bilateraly balanced occlusion refined in the usual manner.

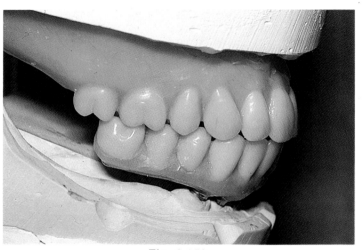

Fig. 3-159

The finished restoration is ready for insertion.

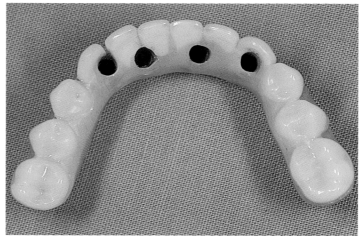

Fig. 3-160

Insertion

As before, the abutments are tightened and thoroughly cleaned. The restoration is then secured into position.

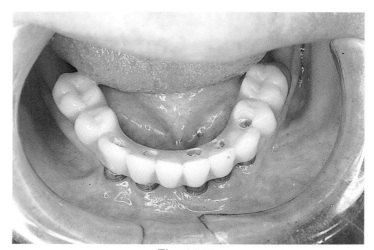

Fig. 3-161

Small cotton pellets are placed over the gold screws, and the access holes are filled with a temporary cement. This allows easy removal of the restoration should an early complication occur. The restoration may need to be removed and cleaned in the first few weeks while hygiene techniques are being perfected.

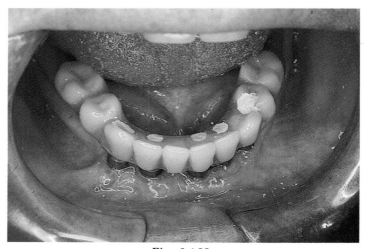

Fig. 3-162

Periapical radiographs are useful to insure proper seating of the abutments and prosthesis. Complaints of pain or discomfort are often indicative of improper seating of the various components.

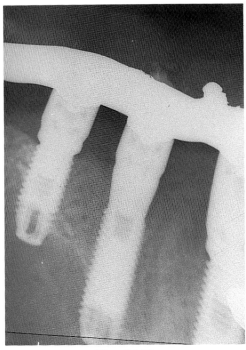

Fig. 3-163

Hygiene/Maintenance

Hygiene instructions are given to the patient. Most helpful is the proxabrush[2], which may be curved to allow for easier lingual access to the abutment cylinders. The end tuft brush is effective in many patients.

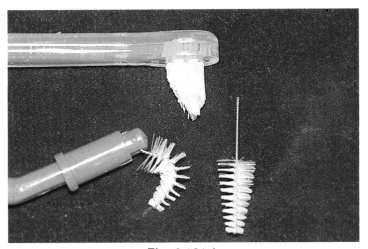

Fig. 3-164,A

The proxabrush² is now designed with a central nylon bristle (b), as opposed to metal, thereby avoiding damage to the titanium abutment.

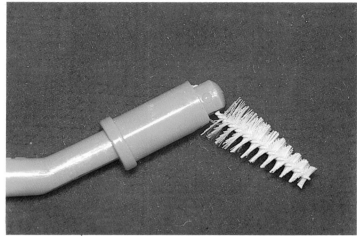

Fig. 3-164,B

The proxabrush² is effective for use on the proximal surfaces of the abutment cylinders (Figs. 3-165,A and B).

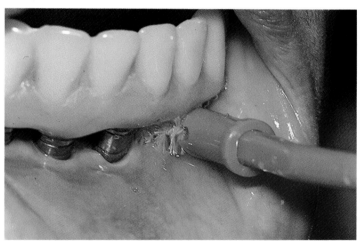

Fig. 3-165,A

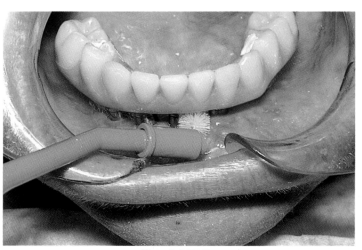

Fig. 3-165,B

An end tuft brush[3] can be adapted to reach the lingual surfaces of the restoration.

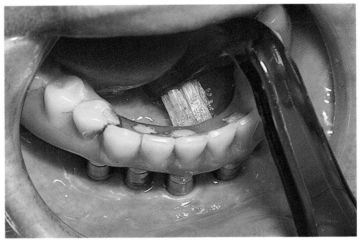

Fig. 3-166

Some patients may be unable to maintain adequate oral hygiene during the first few weeks. The restoration must be removed and cleaned. This problem should be fully exlained to the patient so that he can understand and appreciate the need for better home care.

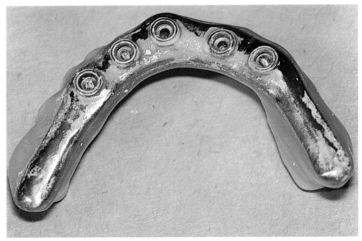

Fig. 3-167

Significant amounts of plaque and calculus can accumulate around the abutment cylinders during this period.

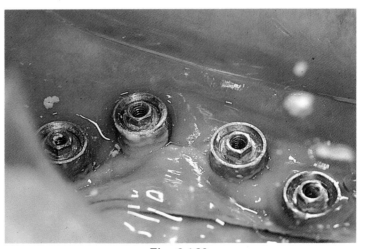

Fig. 3-168

Plastic hygiene instruments have been developed to aid in the removal of debris and calcified deposits around the abutment cylinders. Conventional metal instrumentation would damage the surface of the titanium abutment cylinders and should not be used.

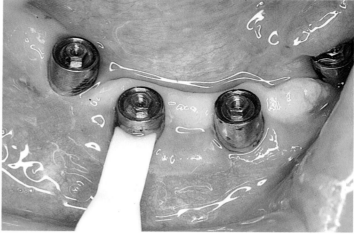

Fig. 3-169

Sealing Screw Access Holes

Once the patient has demonstrated the ability to maintain adequate oral hygiene, the cotton and temporary cement can be replaced with gutta percha covered by a layer of either light-cured or self-curing resin. The patient is placed on a three month recall schedule.

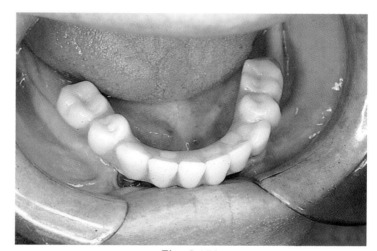

Fig. 3-170

This restoration has been in place for three and one-half years. Oral hygiene and soft tissue health has been excellent.

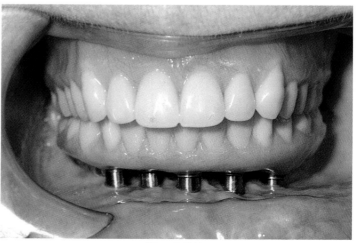

Fig. 3-171

The restoration can provide comfort and function that the patient has not realized for many years. The patient's attitude and quality of life can be affected in a very dramatic fashion.

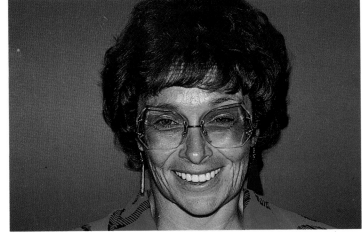

Fig. 3-172

MAXILLARY PROSTHESES

Soft Tissue Considerations

There are significant differences between the maxillary and mandibular arches. The maxillary ridge is often covered by large amounts of keratinized attached mucosa. For this reason, soft tissue complications are not as prevalent as in the mandible.

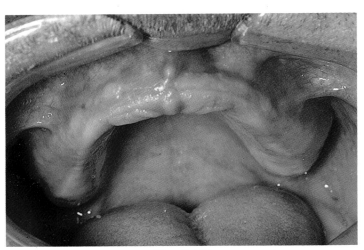

Fig. 3-173

Soft tissue health is more easily maintained around maxillary implants because they are more often encompassed by keratinized attached mucosa.

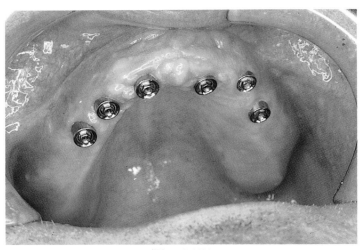

Fig. 3-174

The limiting factor in the maxillary posterior region is the location and morphology of the maxillary sinuses. Even in patients demonstrating minimal to moderate resorption, insufficient amounts of bone may remain below the sinuses to allow fixture placement. Due to the many anatomic variations in sinus size and configuration, it is not unusual that the canine areas (radiopaque markers) are the distal-most positions that maxillary fixtures can be placed.

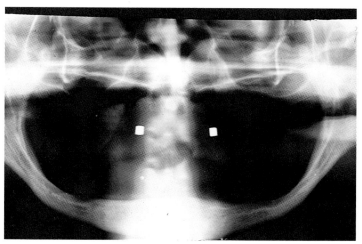

Fig. 3-175

Occlusal Considerations

Due to the inferior quality of maxillary bone compared to mandibular bone, it is recommended that the final prosthesis be cantilevered no more than 10 mm versus 20 mm in the mandible. This may limit the extension of the posterior occlusion in some patients.

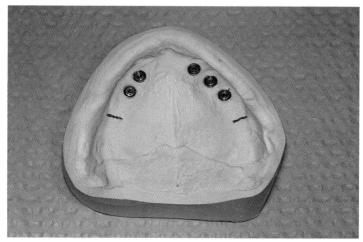

Fig. 3-176

Esthetic Considerations

It would appear that a large maxillary alveolar ridge would be ideal for a bone anchored fixed bridge supported by implants. However, several unacceptable compromises such as esthetics and hygiene access may result if a fixed restoration is employed.

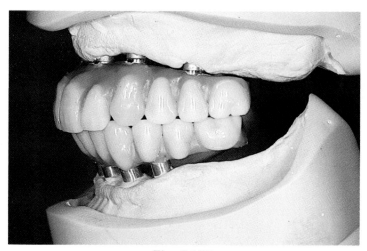

Fig. 3-177

Efforts to cover the open spaces between the final restoration and the alveolar ridge may compromise oral hygiene access.

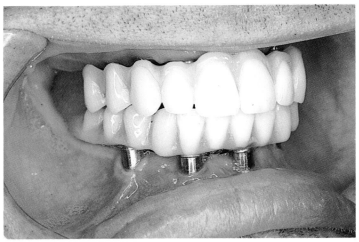

Fig. 3-178

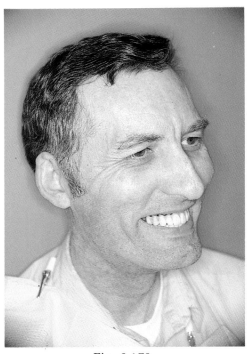

Fig. 3-179

Despite attempts to improve esthetics in the maxillary arch, patients with a high lip line may reveal the abutments and adjacent spaces. In addition, flow of the airstream beneath the restoration may adversely effect speech articulation.

In some patients with moderate resorption and a low upper lip line, there may be adequate space to position the teeth to restore proper esthetics and function, to develop appropriate gingival contours, to maintain adequate space, and to develop appropriate convex tissue surface contours for hygiene access.

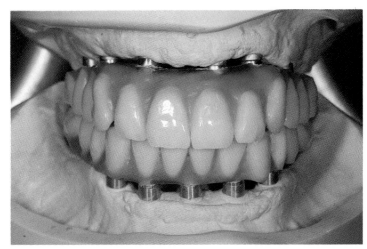

Fig. 3-180

The teeth and denture resin are visible, but the hygienic spaces are usually undetectable in this maxillary fixed bone anchored bridge. Speech articulation may still be compromised initially due to the escape of air beneath the maxillary restoration.

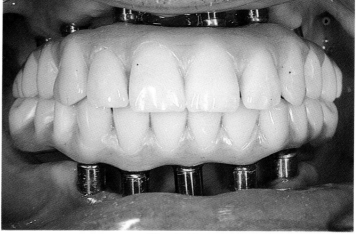

Fig. 3-181

Functional Compromises

This patient complained of compromised upper lip support and experienced difficulty with speech articulation. The arrows illustrate the pathway for air escape during speech. Most patients overcome this functional problem, but in some the airstream must be blocked to enable acceptable speech articulation.

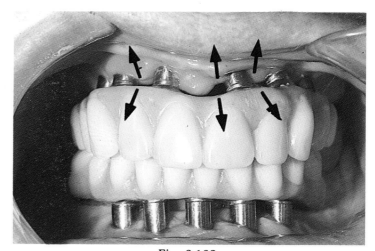

Fig. 3-182

A buccal facade is waxed and processed in acrylic resin and silicone. This removable prosthesis can seal the space between the alveolar ridge and fixed restoration, appropriately directing the airstream over the incisal edges.

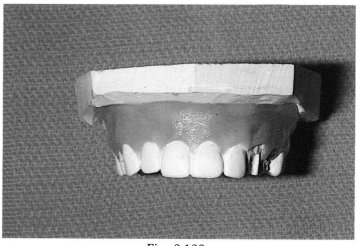

Fig. 3-183

With the facade in place, speech and esthetics are improved. The facade can easily be removed for hygiene.

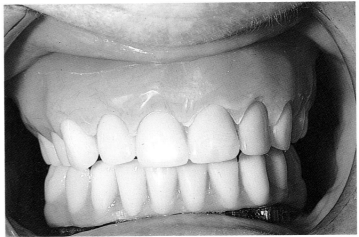

Fig. 3-184

Mandibular facades can also be fabricated for patients concerned about the lack of lip support.

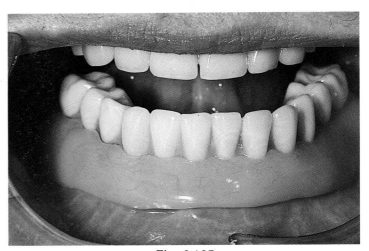

Fig. 3-185

PRODUCT CREDITS

1. Duralay, Reliance Dental Manufacturing Company, Worth, Illinois.
2. Proxabrush, John O. Butler Co., Chicago, Illinois.
3. End Tuft Brush, John O. Butler Co., Chicago, Illinois.

CHAPTER 4   Overlay Prostheses

INTRODUCTION

The use of implant retained and supported removable prostheses, especially in the edentulous mandible, can greatly improve the quality of life for patients who have not been able to function effectively with conventional complete dentures. Many patients would prefer a fixed prosthesis rather than a removable one, but due to anatomic, physiologic, esthetic, or oral hygiene limitations, some patients may only have the option for the latter. Removable overlay dentures offer other distinct advantages: They provide better access for hygiene; the esthetic result is superior; and in many patients it may be the desired means of restoring congenital, traumatic, or surgical defects. The following chapter describes the fabrication and uses of various types of implant-retained overlay prostheses.

INDICATIONS

Satisfying a patient fitted with mandibular complete dentures is a difficult task. There are several important factors critical to a successful result. A large, well-contoured mandibular ridge covered with keratinized attached mucosa will provide appropriate support. Of additional concern is the size and shape of the buccal shelf, tongue position, floor of mouth posture, the patient's ability to control the denture, and the patient's expectations. Compromise of any of the above can lead to impairment in denture function. Use of an implant-supported and retained overlay denture improves function dramatically.

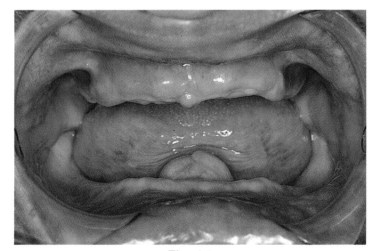

Fig. 4-1

In most edentulous patients it is important to design a complete denture that covers as much tissue bearing surface area as possible. Denture support, stability, and retention will be maximized with this practice.

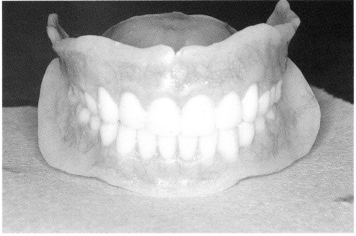

Fig. 4-2

It may be advantageous to allow for removal of the prosthesis to enable the patient to clean directly around the implant abutments. It should not be assumed that patients who present with poor dental compliance will suddenly change their attitude and be able to adequately maintain a fixed bone-anchored prosthesis. If the patient improves their home care, additional implant fixtures can be placed, and a fixed prosthesis can be fabricated at a later time.

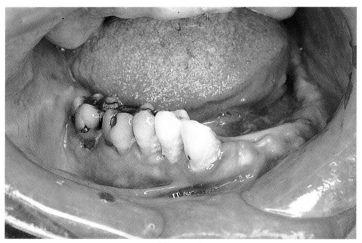

Fig. 4-3

The maxillary arch will usually provide good support for a complete denture, but lateral stability and retention may be compromised in patients with severe resorption. Implant fixtures provide support and stability, and facilitate retention. Masticatory function is thus improved dramatically.

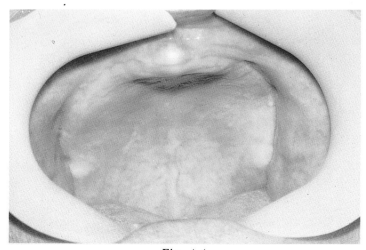

Fig. 4-4

The presence of natural teeth in one arch opposing a complete denture may lead to rapid resorption of the edentulous ridge. The placement of two or more implant fixtures in the edentulous jaw, and fabrication of a removable overlay prosthesis, appears to decrease the risk of resorption.

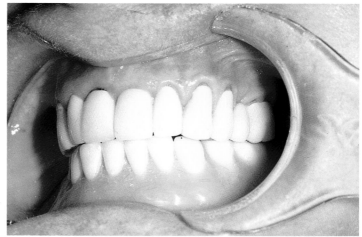

Fig. 4-5

In many edentulous patients, osseointegrated implants are placed in the mandible supporting a fixed prosthesis and opposing an edentulous maxillary arch. This situation is similar to natural dentition opposing a complete denture (Fig. 4-5). The addition of two or more implants in the maxilla supporting an overlay denture may prevent excessive maxillary ridge resorption.

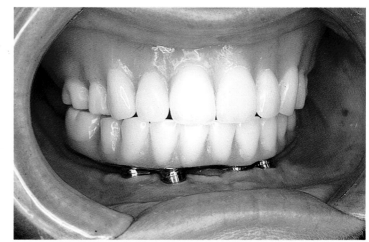

Fig. 4-6

Most patients do well with their maxillary complete denture, but some dislike the presence of the palatal portion of the prosthesis. With the placement of an adequate number of implants, a removable overlay prosthesis lacking palatal coverage can be fabricated.

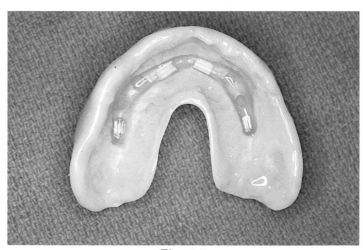

Fig. 4-7

Placement of a fixed bone-anchored maxillary bridge may compromise the esthetic result, and it impairs speech articulation due to the hygienic space necessary between the alveolar ridge and prosthesis (See Chapter 3). An overlay prosthesis eliminates this problem. The denture flange provides the lip support that many patients need, and properly directs the air stream over the incisal edges of the teeth during speech articulation.

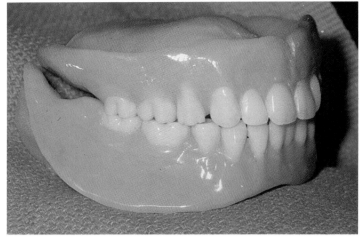

Fig. 4-8

Many elderly patients with cleft palates may have lost the pre-maxillary segment, as well as many teeth, and therefore present with a compromised maxillary foundation area. Removable overlay prostheses are particularly well suited for such patients (Figs. 4-9,A and B).

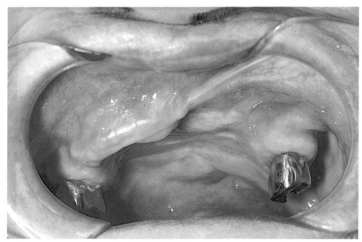

Fig. 4-9,A

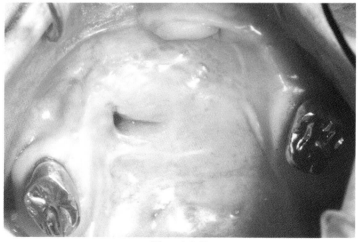

Fig. 4-9,B

Patients who have undergone resections of the maxilla provide a difficult challenge for the restorative dentist. A complete denture with obturator can restore speech and swallowing effectively, but mastication is difficult because of dramatic compromises in retention, stability and support. Implant retained and supported overlay prostheses have provided substantial improvement in function for such patients.

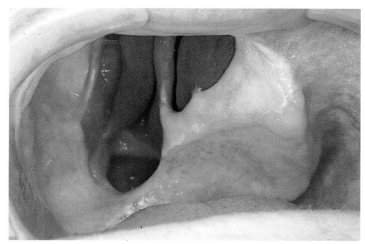

Fig. 4-10

Patients presenting with resections of portions of the mandible secondary to removal of oral tumors can also realize substantial functional benefit from an implant supported and retained overlay prosthesis.

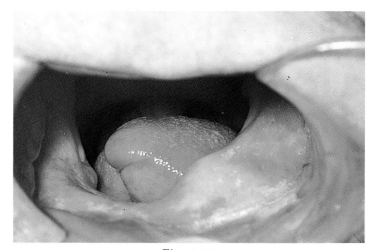

Fig. 4-11

In planning for the placement of two fixtures and fabrication of a removable overlay prosthesis, a thorough intraoral exam is required. The implants will retain the denture, but will also share the occlusal load with the mucoperiosteum.

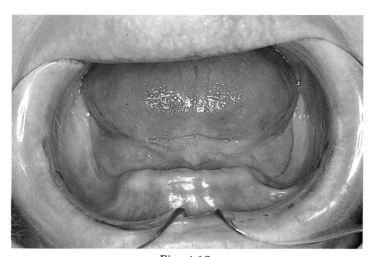

Fig. 4-12

RADIOGRAPHIC ANALYSIS

A panoramic radiograph will help to determine the suitability of the potential bone sites. Ideally, two implants should be placed bilaterally, considering that at a later date additional implants may be desired for fabrication of a fixed bone-anchored bridge.

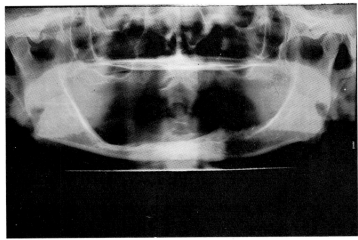

Fig. 4-13

A lateral cephalometric radiograph is useful in determining the buccal-lingual anatomy and ridge angulation in the mandibular anterior region. It is also helpful in determining the density of the bone.

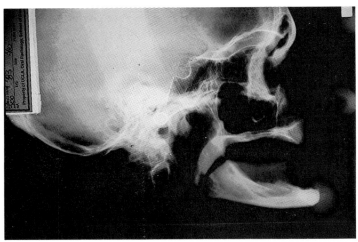

Fig. 4-14

POSTSURGICAL TREATMENT

The techniques used in surgical placement of implant fixtures are identical to those described previously. The surgeon should be reminded that the patient may, at some later date, decide to have additional fixtures placed and a fixed prosthesis fabricated. The location of the two fixtures utilized for the overlay denture must take this into consideration. Following surgery, the patient must go 10-14 days without their denture. When the mucosal incisions are well-healed, the denture is relieved and relined with a tissue conditioner.

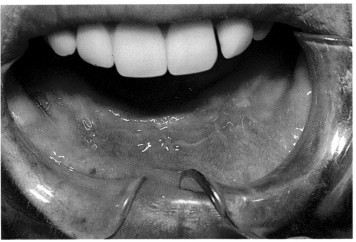

Fig. 4-15

The abutments are connected once osseointegration has occurred. The abutments should project 1-2 mm above the peri-implant tissues. If they extend further, proper positioning of the denture teeth may be compromised.

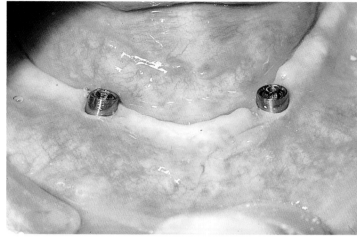

Fig. 4-16

Immediately following abutment connection, the peri-implant tissues are managed in the same manner as discussed in Chapter 3. Oral hygiene must be meticulous, and chlorhexidine gluconate is useful in reducing plaque levels. The placement of healing caps facilitates oral hygiene and promotes healing.

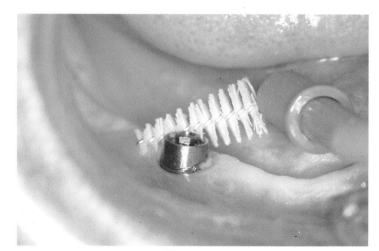

Fig. 4-17

PRELIMINARY IMPRESSIONS

Preliminary impressions can be made once adequate healing has occurred. The abutments are thoroughly cleaned and tightened prior to connecting the tapered impression copings.

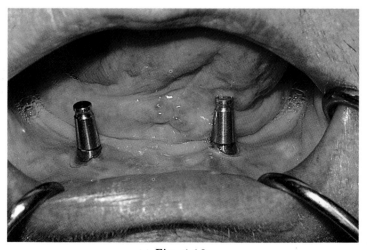

Fig. 4-18

The preliminary irreversible hydrocolloid impression is made with a stock metal tray. When removed, the tapered copings are unscrewed from the abutments and connected to brass analogues. The copings are then inserted back into the impression and the preliminary cast is poured.

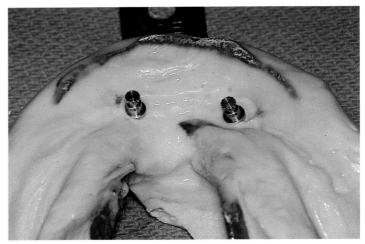

Fig. 4-19

TISSUE BAR FABRICATION

The preliminary cast with the brass analogues in position is now used to fabricate the metal tissue bar.

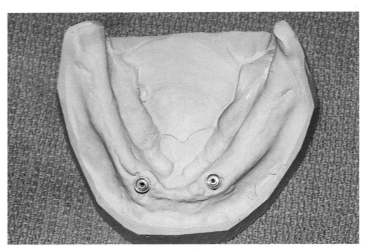

Fig. 4-20

Gold Cylinders

The gold cylinders are placed on the preliminary cast and are connected with guide screws.

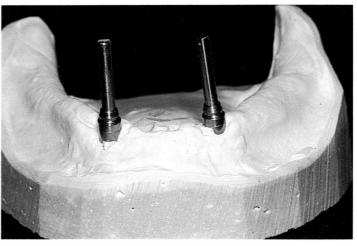

Fig. 4-21

Plastic Pattern

The plastic bar pattern (Fig. 4-22,A) is sectioned and applied to the gold cylinders using cyanoacrylate.

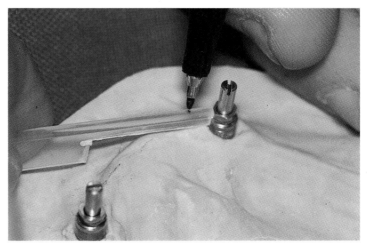

Fig. 4-22,A

The portion of the bar engaged by the retentive clips should be parallel to the axis of rotation of the overlay prosthesis (Fig. 4-22,B). This is difficult to achieve if the implants are placed too posteriorly as the resultant cantilever may be excessive.

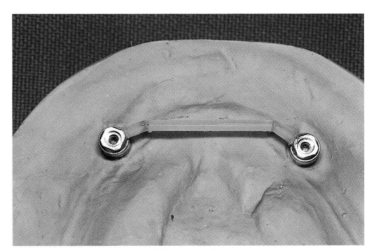

Fig. 4-22,B

When luting the plastic bar pattern to the gold cylinder, care must be taken to avoid flowing wax to its bottom edge.

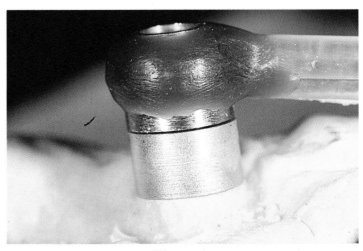

Fig. 4-23

The wax pattern is sprued and invested. A silver palladium alloy was used for casting.

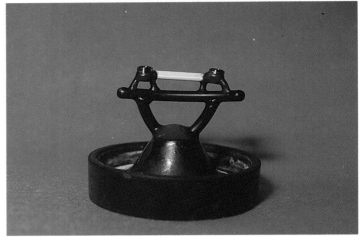

Fig. 4-24

Cast Restoration

The cast tissue bar is finished and polished. The technician must take care to avoid damaging the bottom surface of the gold cylinders.

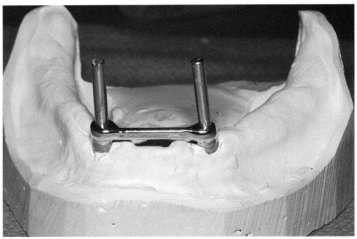

Fig. 4-25

MASTER IMPRESSION

Preliminary Cast Block Out

A master impression tray is now fabricated. The bar and implants must first be blocked out with wax.

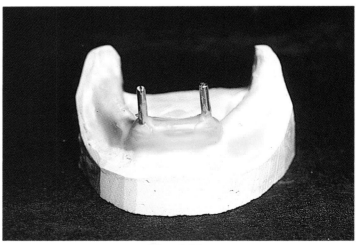

Fig. 4-26

Custom Impression Tray

The completed impression tray is fabricated of tray resin. The tissue bar will be secured to the abutments during the impression with long guide screws and will be removed with the completed impression. It is necessary, therefore, to provide access holes for the long guide screws in the tray.

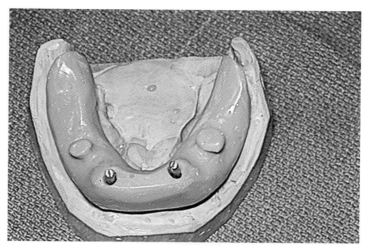

Fig. 4-27

The tissue surface of the impression tray is shown. Note the relief provided for the implants and bar apparatus.

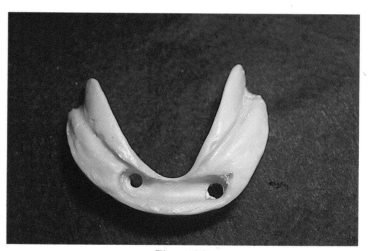

Fig. 4-28

Framework Try-in

Prior to making the master impression, the tissue bar is secured to the implant abutments to verify proper fit. If necessary, the tissue bar is sectioned and soldered prior to making the master impression.

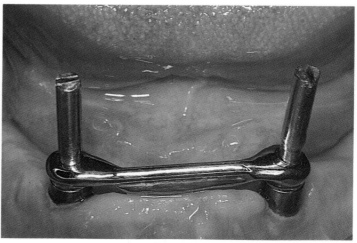

Fig. 4-29

Impression

The final impression, using a border-molded master impression tray, will record the denture bearing surfaces and peripheral extension areas, enhancing support and stability of the definitive prosthesis.

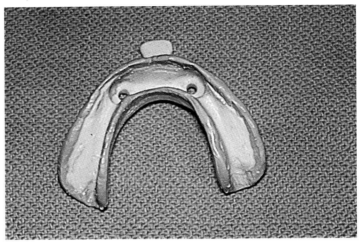

Fig. 4-30

The polysulfide impression has been made. Note that the tissue bar has been incorporated within the impression.

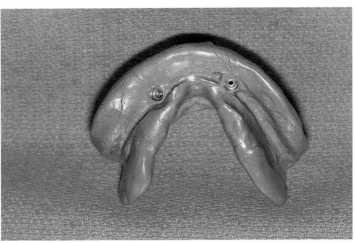

Fig. 4-31

Brass analogues are connected to the gold cylinders of the tissue bar, the impression boxed, and the master cast prepared in the usual manner.

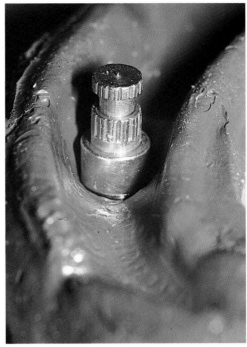

Fig. 4-32

Master Cast

The master cast with the tissue bar is shown ready for denture fabrication.

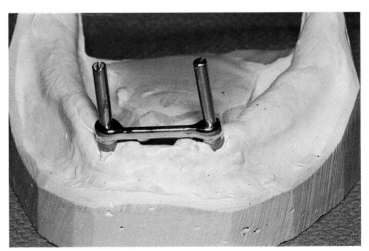

Fig. 4-33

Retentive Clips

The clips (Fig. 4-34,A) and tissue bar (Fig. 4-34,B) are designed and configured to allow for rotation of the overlay prosthesis when a posterior load is applied.

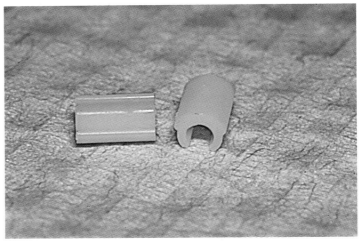

Fig. 4-34,A

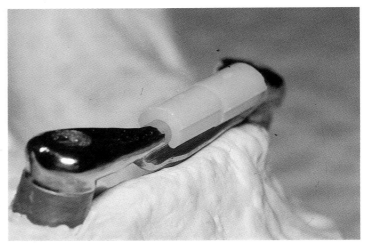

Fig. 4-34,B

CENTRIC RELATION RECORDS

Record Base Fabrication

Record bases are then fabricated. The record base is designed with retentive clips incorporated within it. This provides for a stable and retentive record base and leads to more accurate reproducible centric relation records. The tissue bar and abutments (Figs. 4-35,A and B) should be relieved with wax prior to applying the autopolymerizing acrylic resin to the cast.

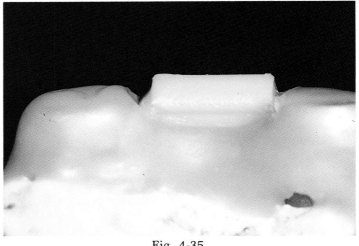

Fig. 4-35

Autopolymerizing acrylic resin is applied to the cast in the usual fashion. Following polymerization, the record base is finished and polished.

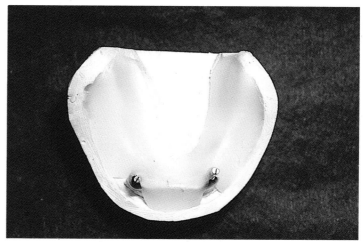

Fig. 4-36

The wax occlusal rim is added. Note the absence of wax over the implants.

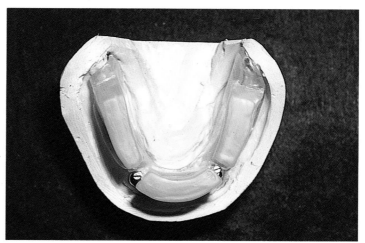

Fig. 4-37

A view of the underside of the record base reveals the retentive clip.

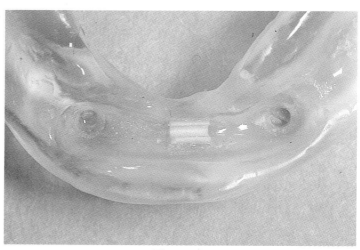

Fig. 4-38

Intraoral Records

An arbitrary hinge axis and a facebow transfer is retrieved, and a centric relation record is made at the appropriate vertical dimension of occlusion. The clip-retained record base improves the accuracy and reproducibility of all records.

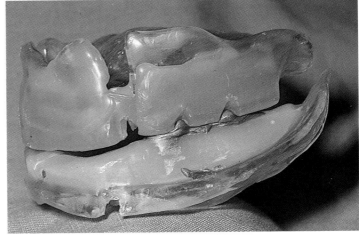

Fig. 4-39

TRIAL DENTURES

Tooth Selection

The centric relation records are transferred to an appropriate articulator. The teeth are selected and wax trial dentures are made. A bilaterally balanced occlusion is recommended, regardless of whether anatomic or nonanatomic posterior teeth are selected.

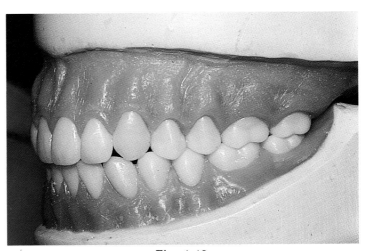

Fig. 4-40

Clinical Try-in

The wax trial dentures are brought to the patient to verify the vertical dimension of occlusion, centric relation, and esthetics. Protrusive and/or lateral records are made.

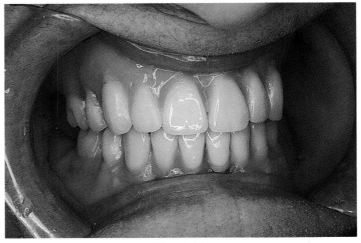

Fig. 4-41

INVESTING AND PROCESSING

Investing

The wax trial dentures are finished and flasked in the usual manner.

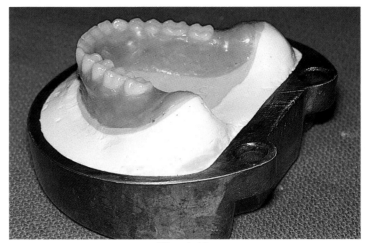

Fig. 4-42

After wax elimination, one side of the flask contains the master cast with brass analogues and the tissue bar. New retention clips, plastic or metal, are placed on the bar so that they will become incorporated into the definitive prosthesis.

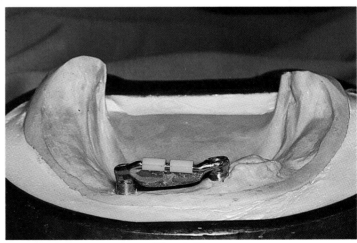

Fig. 4-43

Tissue Bar Block-out

The abutment analogues, tissue bar, and parts of the retentive clips are blocked out with stone to prevent the processing of heat polymerizing acrylic resin in these areas.

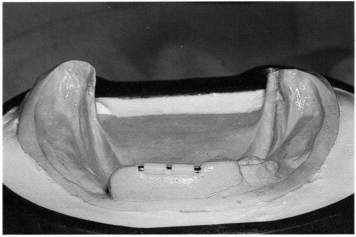

Fig. 4-44

Processing/Finishing

The acrylic resin is processed in the conventional manner. The dentures and casts are placed back on the articulator and equilibrated.

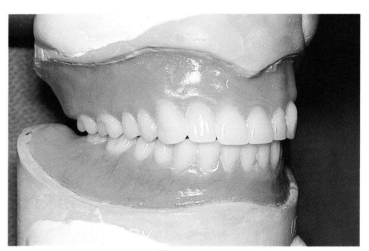

Fig. 4-45

The dentures are removed from the working casts, finished, and polished.

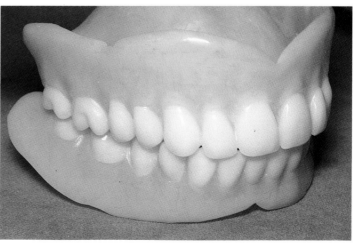

Fig. 4-46

DEFINITIVE RESTORATION

Note the plastic retentive clips imbedded within the denture. This area must be thoroughly cleaned of stone and resin flash. The area adjacent to the clips is inspected carefully, and unwanted debris is removed (Figs. 4-47,A and B).

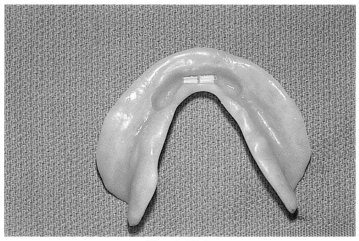

Fig. 4-47,A

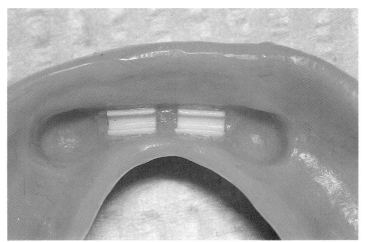

Fig. 4-47,B

Clip Replacement

Plastic clips can be removed easily with a spoon excavator. When necessary, new clips are positioned with the aid of a specially designed instrument. The clips are held in place by mechanical retention.

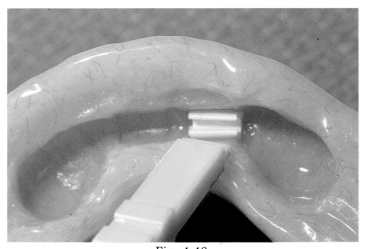

Fig. 4-48

Metal clips may also be used. They are easier to adjust than plastic clips and usually last longer, but they are more difficult to replace.

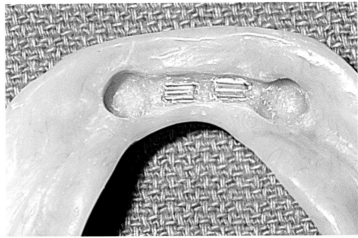

Fig. 4-49

Delivery

The abutments are cleaned and tightened, and the tissue bar secured. The screw access holes may be filled with resin.

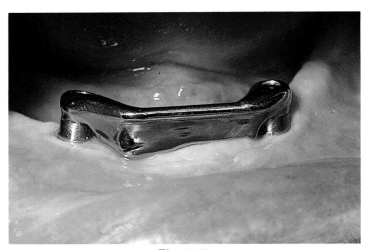

Fig. 4-50

The dentures are delivered in the conventional manner. Pressure indicating paste is used to relieve potential pressure areas. Disclosing wax is used to evaluate the extensions.

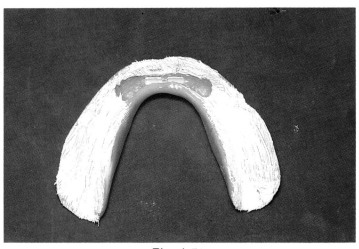

Fig. 4-51

Clinical Remount

The vertical dimension of occlusion is verified, and a new centric relation record is made. The prostheses are remounted on the articulator and the occlusion is refined. It is important to achieve proper centric relation contacts and bilateral balanced occlusion.

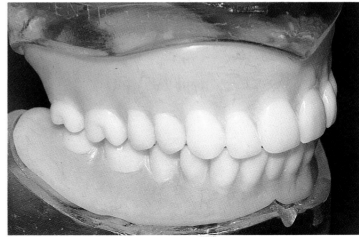

Fig. 4-52

Hygiene

Oral hygiene procedures are reviewed with the patient. Various aids can be utilized, although the proxabrush appears to be the most suitable for this type of restoration.

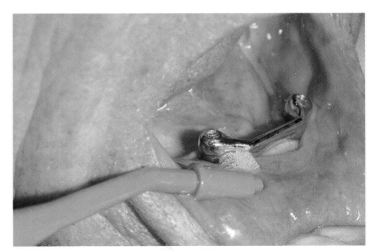

Fig. 4-53

The dentures are delivered, and post-insertion instructions are provided.

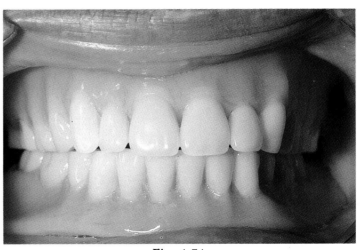

Fig. 4-54

Patients with implant-retained removable overlay dentures report remarkable improvement and satisfaction with their new prostheses. This method of treatment should be kept in mind when evaluating all edentulous and partially edentulous patients. Forces generated during mastication can be improved dramatically with this prosthesis *(Carr et al, 1987)*.

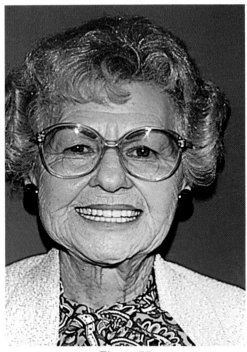

Fig. 4-55

MAXILLARY RESTORATIONS

Two Fixtures

While most patients function well with a complete maxillary denture, some with resorbed maxillary ridges may present with compromised denture stability. Two implant fixtures can be placed to facilitate denture retention and stability, as well as to prevent excessive resorption when opposing either natural dentition or a mandibular fixed bone anchored bridge.

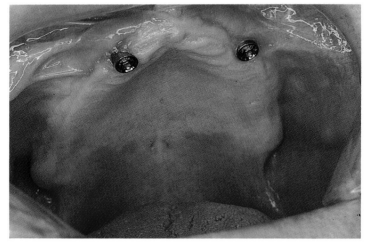

Fig. 4-56

The tissue bar seen here follows the contours of the alveolar process. The tissue bar is designed to accept the anterior occlusal loads. The posterior loads are absorbed by the mucoperiosteum of the denture support areas.

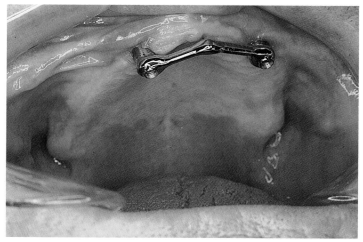

Fig. 4-57

The tissue surface and peripheral extensions of the prosthesis are similar to that of a conventional maxillary denture except for the placement of retentive clips (Fig. 4-58,A). Support is provided jointly by the implants and the mucoperiosteum.

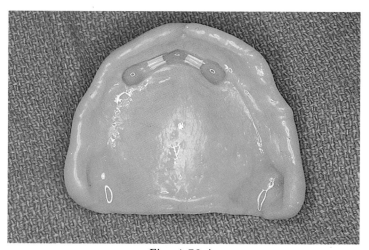

Fig. 4-58,A

Figure 4-58,B illustrates a more favorable tissue bar because the bar is designed such that when posterior occlusal loads are applied, the bar is parallel to the axis of rotation of the prosthesis.

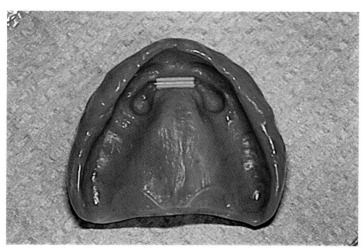

Fig. 4-58,B

The completed maxillary removable overlay prosthesis opposes a mandibular fixed bone anchored bridge.

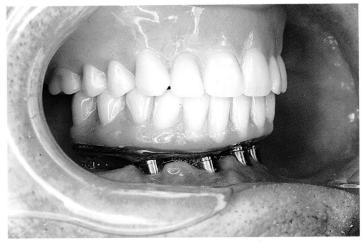

Fig. 4-59

Four Fixtures

Some patients feel uncomfortable wearing a prosthesis which covers the palatal vault. With the placement of four or more implants, the fixtures can now be utilized to support and retain a ''vaultless'' maxillary overlay denture.

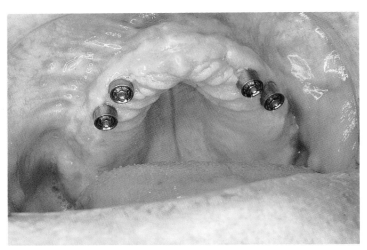

Fig. 4-60

A tissue bar anchored by four fixtures can be cantilevered a short distance posterior to the distal abutments. The prosthesis extends posteriorly to cover the maxillary tuberosity. Support is shared between the mucoperiosteum in this region and the four implants.

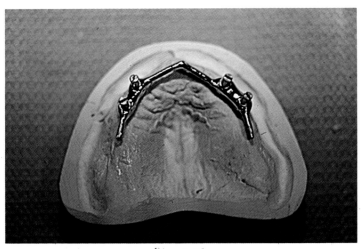

Fig. 4-61

The tissue bar is connected to the four implants. Anteriorly, it follows the configuration of the alveolar process.

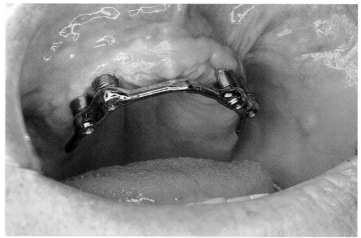

Fig. 4-62

The completed prosthesis is shown. Support is shared by both the alveolar process posteriorly and the implant supported tissue bar. In this patient, the posterior metal clips were adjusted to be non-retentive, and are designed to load the tissue bar. The anterior plastic clips provide more than adequate retention.

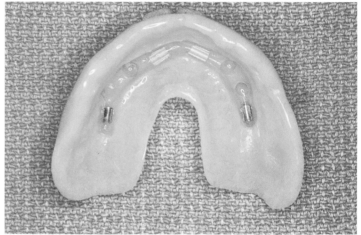

Fig. 4-63

The completed maxillary removable overlay prosthesis in position opposes natural dentition. Particular care was taken to reshape the opposing natural mandibular dentition and adjust the occlusal plane so that a bilateral balanced occlusion could be achieved.

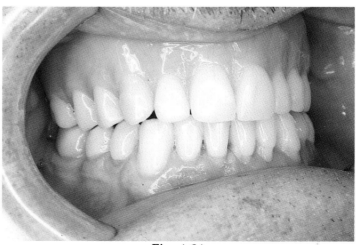

Fig. 4-64

Six Fixtures

The placement of six implants in the maxilla and the fabrication of a tissue bar allows the prosthesis to be completely implant-supported.

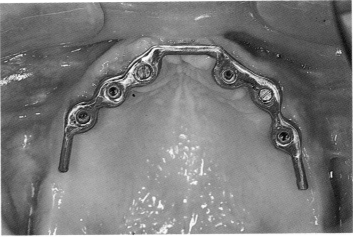

Fig. 4-65

Due to minimal maxillary ridge resorption, a low-profile tissue bar was necessary for appropriate placement of denture teeth.

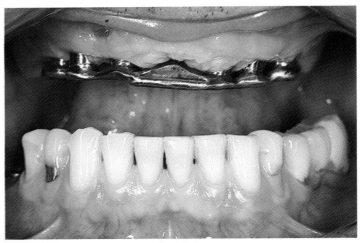

Fig. 4-66

Three plastic clips are incorporated into the tissue surface of the prosthesis and provide retention.

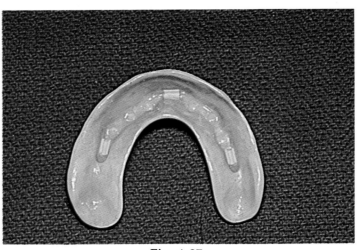

Fig. 4-67

The implants and tissue bar are used for support, and it is not necessary to cover the palatal vault. However, it is necessary to extend the prosthesis to the soft tissues to prevent food impaction.

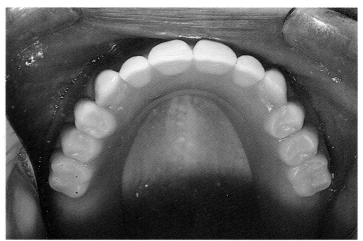

Fig. 4-68

The buccal flange of this "fixed/detachable" overlay prosthesis provides several functional and esthetic advantages over a fixed restoration. Removal of the prosthesis allows the patient easy access for oral hygiene around the implants and tissue bar.

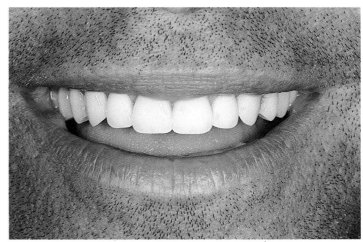

Fig. 4-69

In instances where four or more implants are used to support and retain an overlay prosthesis, such as this mandibular restoration, there is the likelihood that the tissue bar may interfere with the proper position of denture teeth. Wax trial dentures, therefore, should be completed before the bar is designed.

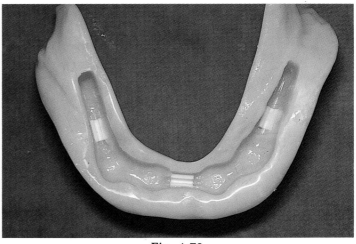

Fig. 4-70

A matrix is made from the trial denture and the tissue bar is designed accordingly. This method is similar to that used in the fabrication of the metal framework for an edentulous fixed bone-anchored bridge.

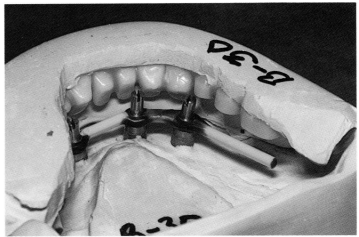

Fig. 4-71

With the matrix and teeth in position, note that sufficient space exists for the denture over the tissue bar.

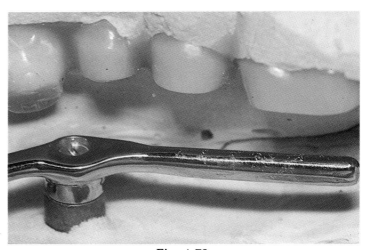

Fig. 4-72

The finished restoration is retained and supported by the four implants and tissue bar. The support for the lower lip necessary in some patients can be developed with the denture flange.

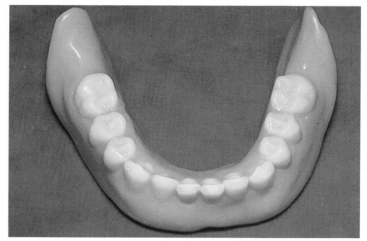

Fig. 4-73

The completed prostheses enables the patient to function as efficiently as with a fixed bone-anchored bridge (Fig. 4-74,A).

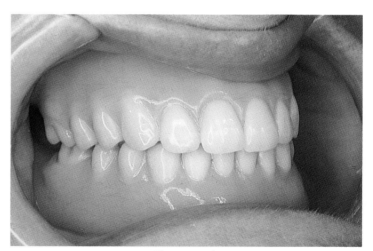

Fig. 4-74,A

In addition the prostheses can be removed and oral hygiene access to implant surfaces improves dramatically (Fig. 4-74,B).

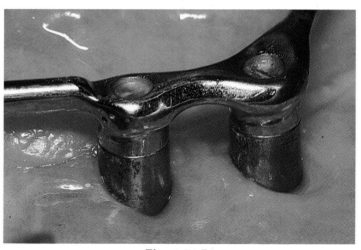

Fig. 4-74,B

CLEFT PALATE PROSTHESES

Patients with cleft palate often wear removable prostheses which not only replace missing teeth, but also restore the vertical dimension of occlusion, occlusal plane, intraoral and facial contours, as well as palatopharyngeal function.

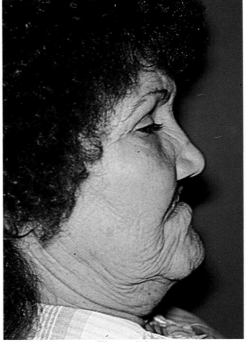

Fig. 4-75

The few remaining teeth are often compromised due to the fact that they have been required to support and retain a large dental prosthesis for many years.

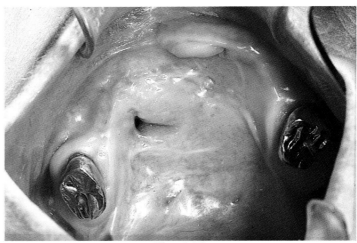

Fig. 4-76

Osseointegrated implants can be placed to provide support and retention for a removable overlay prosthesis and help to preserve the remaining teeth. The limiting factor with these patients is the amount of remaining bone available for fixture placement.

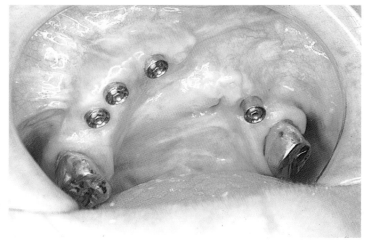

Fig. 4-77

A tissue bar joins two fixtures together, and will be utilized for support and retention of the final prosthesis. Since the lone standing implant was short and was separated from those on the opposite side by the cleft, additional healing time was required prior to loading. Delayed use of implants in poor-quality maxillary bone beds may be desirable in some patients. Note that in this patient one fixture failed to osseointegrate. It was subsequently removed.

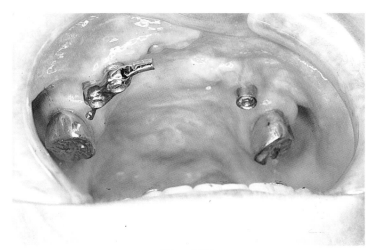

Fig. 4-78

The male portion of an O-SO[1] attachment was connected to the lone standing fixture.

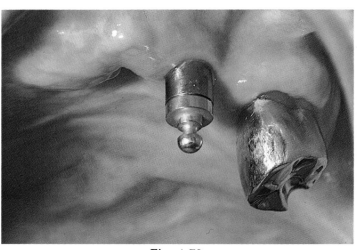

Fig. 4-79

The male O-SO[1] attachment screws into the abutment screw. The elastic ring of the female attachment provides a firm fit onto the male. The white or red elastic ring is positioned within a metal collar.

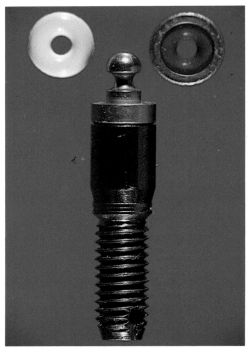

Fig. 4-80

The female attachment, incorporated within a metal collar, fits over the male portion.

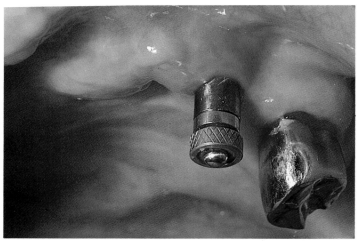

Fig. 4-81

The metal collar encompassing the elastic female ring is secured to the prosthesis with autopolymerizing acrylic resin. This procedure can also be accomplished by placing the male and female attachments on the master cast prior to packing and processing the prosthesis.

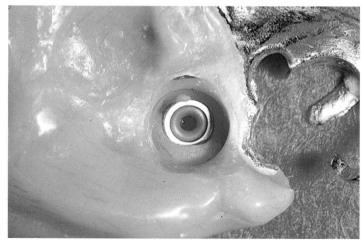

Fig. 4-82

The tissue surface of the prosthesis now contains the plastic clips used for attachment onto the tissue bar, and also the female O-SO[1] attachment that connects to the male.

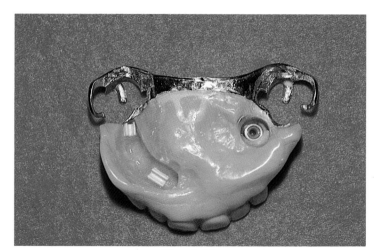

Fig. 4-83

The final removable overlay partial denture is retained by the implants, providing a stable, retentive, and well supported prosthesis.

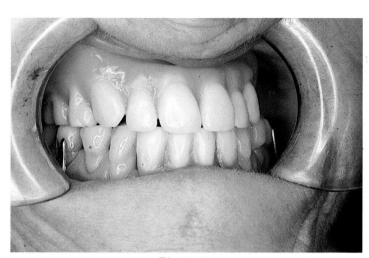

Fig. 4-84

MAXILLARY OBTURATOR PROSTHESES

Patients who have undergone surgical maxillary resections for removal of oral and/or paranasal sinus neoplasms may have significant functional impairment. As in the case of cleft palate patients, large restorations are often necessary to replace the missing intraoral structures. The size and weight of these prostheses is such that they often have detrimental effects on the remaining dentition. If few or no maxillary teeth remain, the patient's ability to function with a prosthesis designed to obturate a large maxillary defect is compromised.

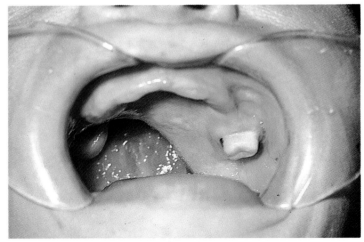

Fig. 4-85

Osseointegrated implant fixtures can provide retention, stability, and support for these large maxillary obturators. Four implants have been placed in this patient who had lost a significant portion of hard and soft palate following resection of an adenoid cystic carcinoma.

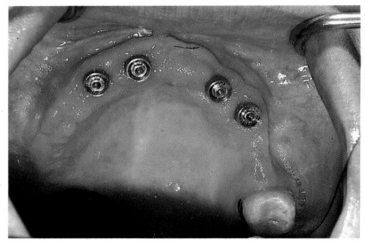

Fig. 4-86

Fabrication of a tissue bar and removable overlay prosthesis is the treatment of choice since a fixed bone-anchored bridge would fail to restore the surgical defect and the palatopharyngeal deficit.

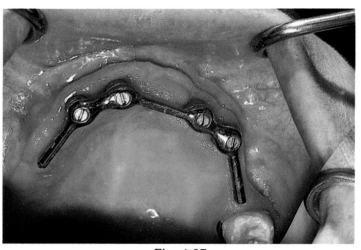

Fig. 4-87

The tissue surface of the prosthesis with the retentive clips in place is shown. Note the obturator portion which restores the palatopharyngeal deficit.

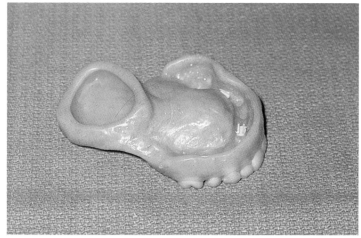

Fig. 4-88

Patients who have previously experienced difficulty in achieving satisfactory function with large maxillary obturators have demonstrated dramatic improvement because of the stability, retention and support provided by an implant supported overlay prosthesis. Speech and swallowing are restored to normal and mastication is dramatically improved.

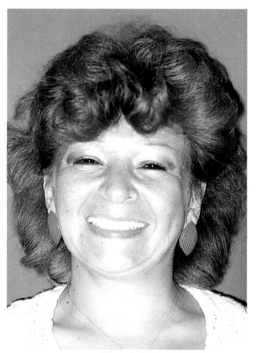

Fig. 4-89

MANDIBULAR RESECTION

Edentulous patients who have undergone mandibular resection for oral cavity tumors present with severe functional impairment. The conventional mandibular resection denture provides limited stability, support, and retention. The use of osseointegrated implants enables fabrication of implant retained and supported overlay prostheses, dramatically improving function in these patients. In this patient, the left body of the mandible has been resected. Two implants were placed and a tissue bar fabricated.

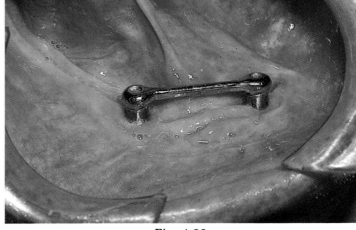

Fig. 4-90

Intraoral records are extremely difficult to make in edentulous patients with mandibular resections due to rotation and deviation of the mandible. The implant-retained record base aids in the recording of maxillo-mandibular relationships (Figs. 4-91,A and B).

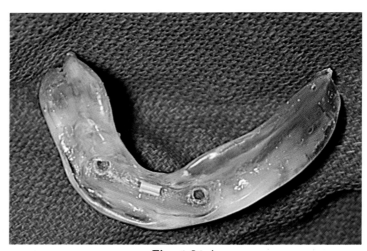

Fig. 4-91,A

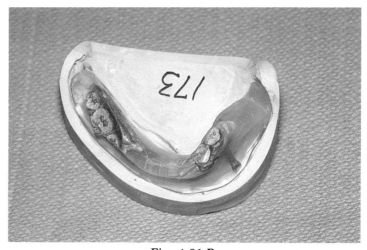

Fig. 4-91,B

The tissue surface of the mandibular prosthesis contains retentive clips.

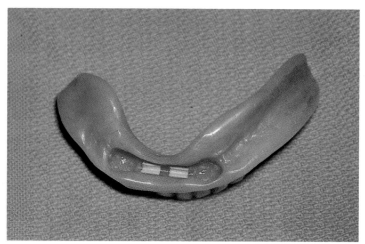

Fig. 4-92

The definitive final overlay prosthesis is extremely stable, well supported and retentive, enabling the patient to function at levels far beyond those previously achieved.

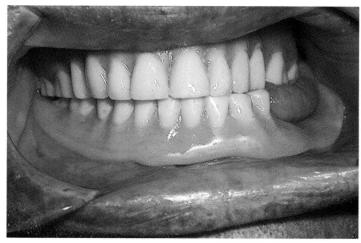

Fig. 4-93

The benefits extend far beyond the realm of intraoral function for this patient.

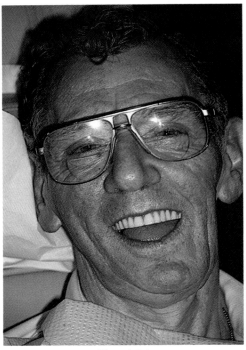

Fig. 4-94

EXTRAORAL APPICATIONS

Smaller (3 to 4 mm) titanium implants can be utilized for the retention of extraoral prosthesis. A flange (Fig. 4-95,A) on the fixture prevents excessive penetration through the thin cranial bones during placement (Fig. 4-95,B).

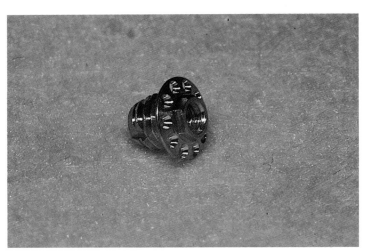

Fig. 4-95,A

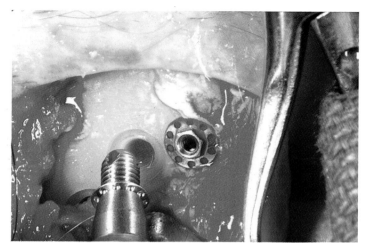

Fig. 4-95,B

Implant fixtures are utilized in this patient to retain an ear prosthesis, eliminating the need for skin adhesives.

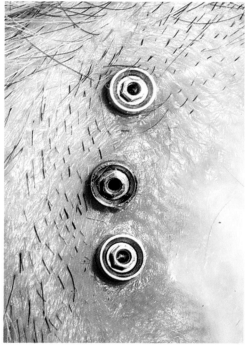

Fig. 4-96

This tissue bar utilizes magnets and clips for the retention of the ear prosthesis (Figs. 4-97,A and B).

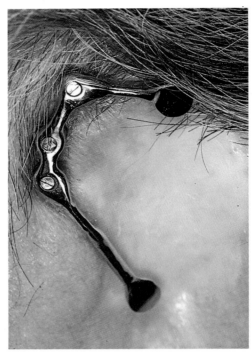

Fig. 4-97,A

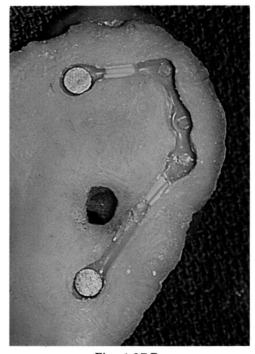

Fig. 4-97,B

The retention of the definitive ear prosthesis is dramatically improved.

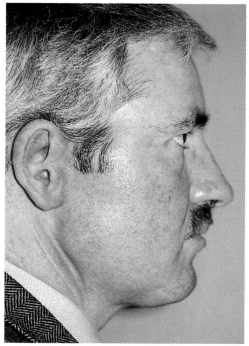

Fig. 4-98

In this rhinectomy defect, an implant fixture has been placed and a tissue bar fabricated with magnets.

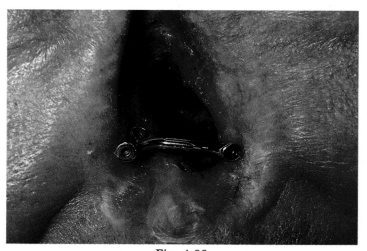

Fig. 4-99

Two magnets are imbedded within the nasal prosthesis (Fig. 4-100,A).

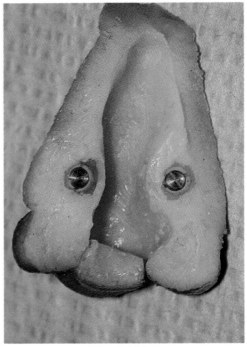

Fig. 4-100,A

These magnets retain the prosthesis (Fig 4-100,B).

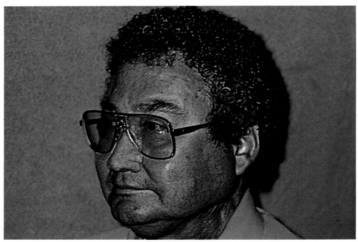

Fig. 4-100,B

Two implants have been placed in the superior orbital rim of this patient who had previously undergone a radical maxillectomy and orbital exenteration (Fig. 4-101,A).

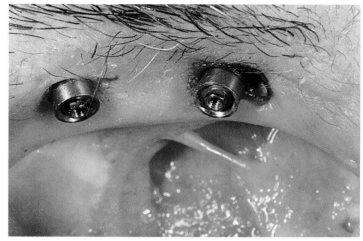

Fig. 4-101,A

A tissue bar with magnets has been attached to the implants (Fig. 4-101,B).

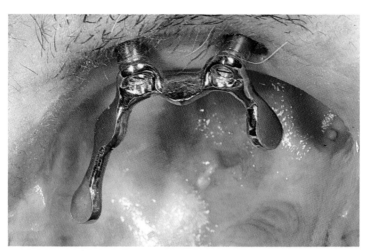

Fig. 4-101,B

Magnets were incorporated within the obturator (Fig. 4-102,A).

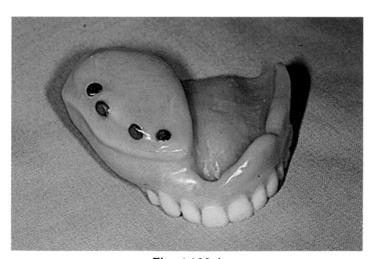

Fig. 4-102,A

The magnetic connection between the obturator and the orbital prosthesis improves retention and stability of the complete denture-obturator prosthesis (Fig. 4-102,B).

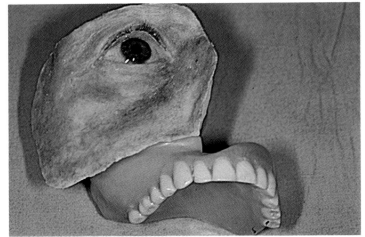

Fig. 4-102,B

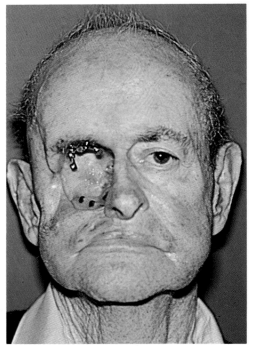

Fig. 4-103,A

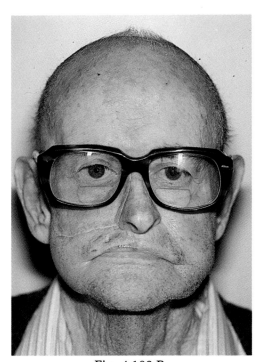

Fig. 4-103,B

With the tissue bar and obturator in position (Fig. 4-103,A), the definitive prosthesis is stabilized (Fig. 4-103,B).

REFERENCES

1. Carr, A., Laney, W.: Maximum occlusal force levels in patients with osseointegrated oral implant prostheses and patients with complete dentures. Int. J. Oral & Max. Implants 2:2, 101-108, 1987.

PRODUCT CREDITS

1. Attachments International, San Mateo, California.

CHAPTER 5   Implant-Supported
Fixed Partial Dentures

INTRODUCTION

The Branemark implant system has been used extensively in the treatment of partially edentulous patients. This patient population is more variable than the edentulous group, and careful diagnosis, treatment planning, and communication among the restorative/surgical team becomes increasingly important. The location and angulation of fixture placement is critical in the partially edentulous patient. Anatomic limitations also play a greater role in the treatment of this group, especially when the placement of posterior implant fixtures is desired. Single tooth restorations, obtaining acceptable esthetic results, and inadequate interocclusal space have posed interesting and difficult challenges for the restorative/surgical team. There are also many unanswered questions concerning treatment of the partially edentulous patient with regard to load carrying capacity, occlusal materials, occlusal schemes, cantilevering, and the interrelationship of the two different support mechanisms (PDL vs direct bone interface). The following chapter attempts to address these and other issues. Conventional restorative techniques, as well as recent developments such as the "UCLA" abutment, will be discussed.

DIAGNOSTIC PROCEDURES

Considerations

This patient presents with a simple restorative problem. While the remaining dentition and restorations are in good condition, a three unit implant-supported fixed partial denture is needed in the mandibular arch due to the length of the edentulous span. Note that the partially edentulous patient will usually present with adequate amounts of attached keratinized tissue in the edentulous areas, resulting in fewer soft tissue complications.

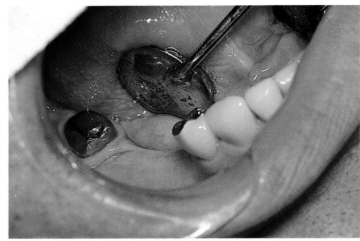

Fig. 5-1

This patient presents with multiple missing and compromised teeth. The diagnosis and treatment planning must include not only the replacement of the missing teeth, but also an assessment of the remaining dentition. The restorative phase of treatment will require a determination of the proper vertical dimension of occlusion, establishing an appropriate occlusal plane and occlusal scheme, restoring the existing teeth, and replacing the missing ones.

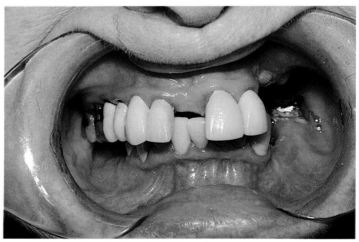

Fig. 5-2

Limited occlusal space is often of concern in the partially edentulous patient due to minimal resorption at the edentulous site and the presence of opposing dentiton. Esthetics will also be a prime factor in the restoration of this patient; for implant position and angulation will directly effect the esthetic result.

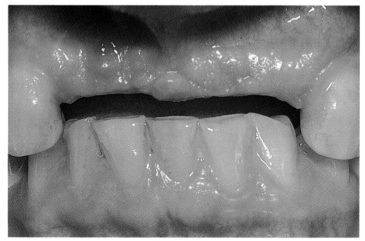

Fig. 5-3

The occlusal load placed on the implant restoration depends upon the nature of the residual dentition. For example, Figure 5-4,A illustrates a patient with a periodontally sound canine with sufficient vertical overlap to allow for tooth-born anterior guidance. The posterior implant-supported fixed restoration can be designed with centric only contacts. Most of the occlusal load can then be directed along the long axis of the implant.

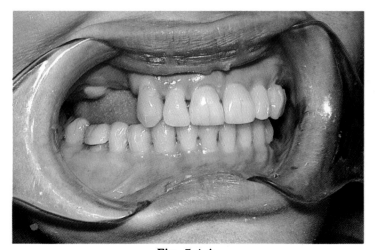

Fig. 5-4,A

In Figure 5-4,B the dentition distal to the right lateral incisor is missing and therefore the implant supported restoration will be exposed to both vertical and horizontal forces. It should be emphasized that it is unclear how well maxillary posterior implants can tolerate these types of occlusal loads.

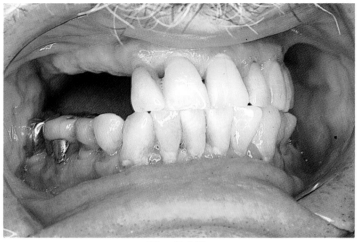

Fig. 5-4,B

Recent technical developments have allowed for fabrication of esthetic and functional single tooth implant-supported restorations. During treatment planning the clinician therefore must consider the status of adjacent natural teeth.

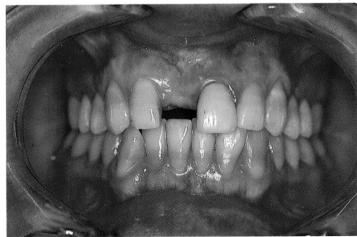

Fig. 5-5

Radiographs

When evaluating a patient for the placement of implant fixtures, a panoramic radiograph is used to determine the approximate quantity and quality of remaining bone. Location of the inferior alveolar nerve and mental foramen is critical. This radiograph appears to reveal an adequate amount of bone available.

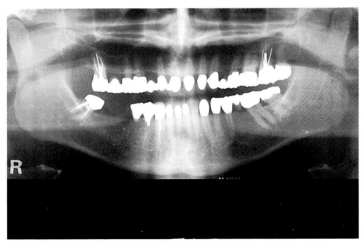

Fig. 5-6

The maxillary sinus is the limiting factor when considering a patient for maxillary posterior implants. A minimum of 10 mm of bone appears to be required for implant placement. It must be remembered that the density of the maxillary cancellous bone is considerably less than that of the mandible, especially in the tuberosity regions.

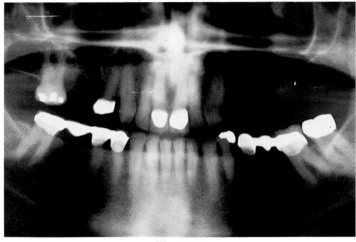

Fig. 5-7

Diagnostic Casts

Diagnostic casts are required in the treatment of all partially edentulous patients. They should be mounted on an appropriate articulator with the use of an arbitrary hinge axis location and facebow transfer and centric relation records.

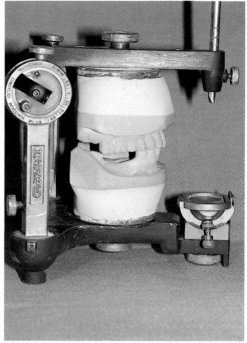

Fig. 5-8

A diagnostic wax-up is prepared on the mounted casts. In this patient, the vertical dimension of occlusion, occlusal plane, and condition of the remaining teeth are acceptable. A preliminary panoramic radiograph (Fig. 5-6) has revealed that adequate bone quantity is probably available for the placement of implants in the edentulous area. The restoration planned will be a fixed partial denture retained and supported by two implant fixtures. The purpose of the diagnostic wax-up is to determine tooth location and optimal fixture placement. The cast is marked at the proposed implant sites.

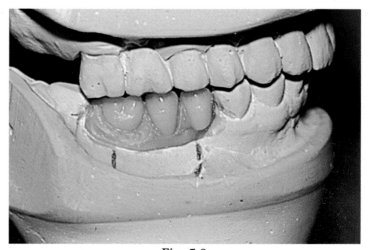

Fig. 5-9

This diagnostic wax-up has been developed for a patient requiring a full mouth rehabilitation (Fig. 5-2). The vertical dimension of occlusion and the occlusal plane are being reconfigured, and the missing teeth replaced. The implant-supported restorations are represented by denture teeth. The initial panoramic radiograph revealed a limited amount of bone in the left posterior maxilla, preventing ideal implant placement. The diagnostic wax-up is thus terminated posteriorly.

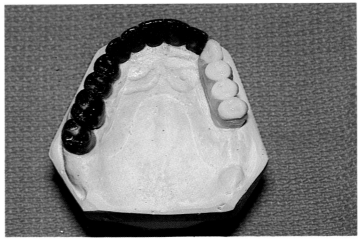

Fig. 5-10

The diagnostic wax-up of the mandibular arch also reflects the limitations seen on the panoramic radiograph. The amount of available bone on the right side is limited by the inferior alveolar nerve and can therefore receive only one implant fixture.

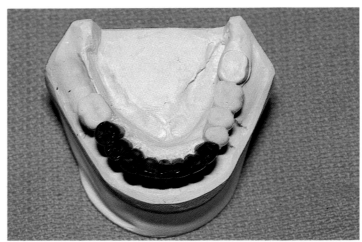

Fig. 5-11

Once the implant location has been determined, the denture teeth are removed and the proposed sites are marked on the crest of the alveolar ridge. This cast is used to fabricate a stent that will be utilized for additional diagnostic radiographs.

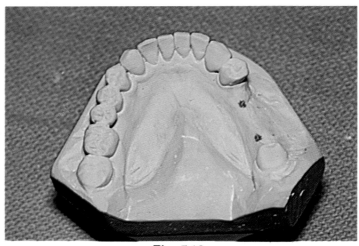

Fig. 5-12

Diagnostic Stents

Sta-guard[1] mouthguard material is vacuum-formed to the diagnostic cast and trimmed appropriately.

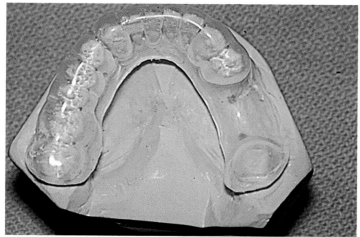

Fig. 5-13

With the stent on the cast, holes are drilled directly over the implant location marks.

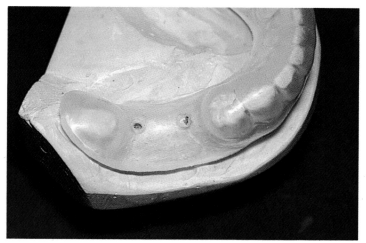

Fig. 5-14

Ball bearings are placed in the stent corresponding to the desired locations for implant placement. It is best to use different sizes of ball bearings in each location.

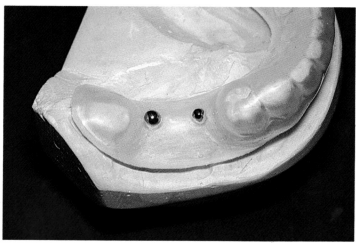

Fig. 5-15

The stent containing ball bearings is placed intraorally, and a panoramic radiograph is made. The ball bearings indicate the proposed implant locations and allows radiographic examination of the proper sites. The panoramic x-ray unit, as it rotates around the patient, does not follow a path directly parallel with the mandible. For this reason, the ratio of distortion differs from point to point and cannot be easily calculated at each individual site. Therefore, the panoramic radiograph does not provide the necessary accuracy needed when considering placement of implant fixtures over the inferior alveolar nerve.

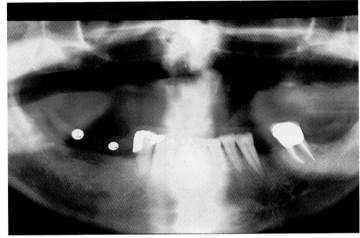

Fig. 5-16

Tomograms

Tomograms are taken with the stent in position. These radiographs show the body of the mandible in cross section. The sections are made at various levels anterior-posteriorly. When the image of the ball bearing is clearly defined, the plane directly through the center of that particular ball bearing is being visualized. Different sizes of ball bearings are utilized when evaluating more than one proposed implant site.

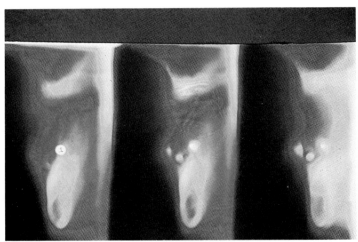

Fig. 5-17

This radiograph shows the ball bearing in focus. An implant fixture has been proposed for this site. The alveolar ridge and mandibular canal are outlined; the magnification calculated; and the exact anatomic dimensions determined.

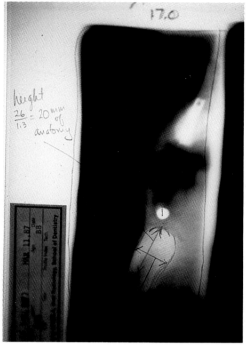

Fig. 5-18

Tomograms are also useful in the posterior maxillary areas for evaluating the available bone and morphology of the maxillary sinus.

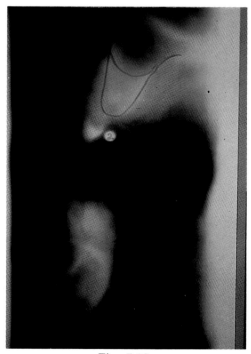

Fig. 5-19

CAT scans provide diagnostic information similar to that from tomograms, but at much greater expense. Another disadvantage is that dental restorations often distort the imaging.

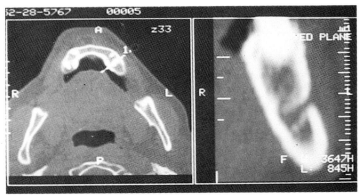

Fig. 5-20

Sugical Stents

By removing the ball bearings, the stent may also be used surgically to aid in correct positioning of the implant fixtures. With the soft tissue flaps reflected and the stent in place, a bur can be used to mark the crest of the ridge at the desired implant sites. The stent is removed and site preparation continues, A disadvantage of a surgical stent designed in this way is that it does not help the operator obtain the proper angulation of the implant fixture (Figs. 5-21,A and B).

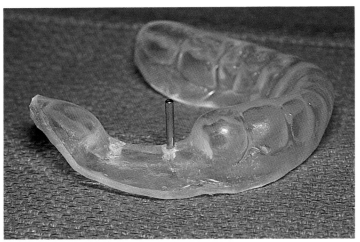

Fig. 5-21,A

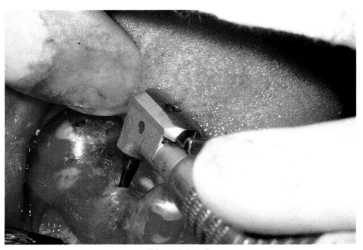

Fig. 5-21,B

The preferred type of surgical stent contains denture teeth and clear acylic resin.

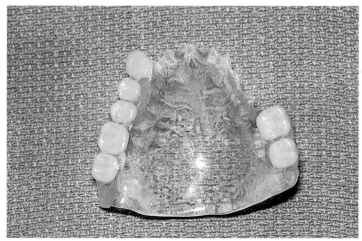

Fig. 5-22

In order to use the stent during surgery, it must be trimmed as shown. The surgical incision is usually made in the buccal vestibule and the flap reflected lingually or palatally. To seat the stent at surgery, the palatal portion must be removed so as not to interfere with the soft tissue flap. With the stent in place, the implant sites can be prepared. The remaining facial shells of the denture teeth serve as guides for proper implant location and angulation.

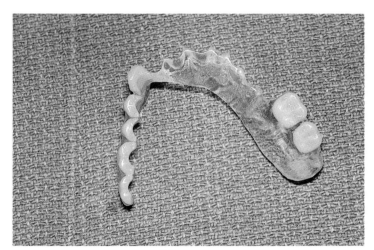

Fig. 5-23

The surgical procedures for implant site preparation and fixture placement are carried out in the usual manner. Proper implant location and angulation are particularly important in the partially edentulous patient.

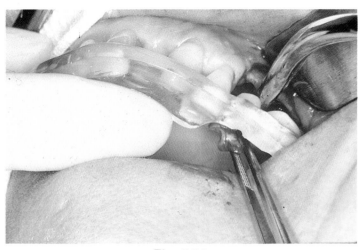

Fig. 5-24

PROVISIONAL RESTORATIONS

Removable Provisionals

If the patient has been wearing a removable prosthesis, it must not be worn for a period of 10-14 days following surgery. After initial healing, the removable prosthesis must be generously relieved and lined with a tissue conditioner (Figs. 5-25,A and B).

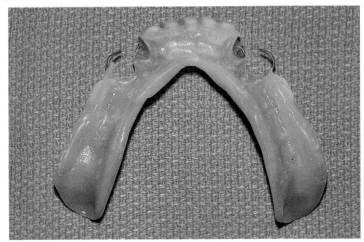

Fig. 5-25,A

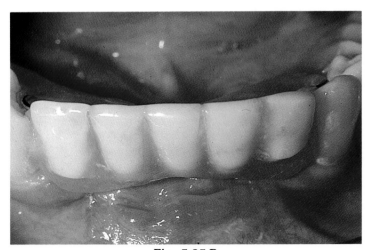

Fig. 5-25,B

Fixed Provisionals

A provisional fixed partial denture may be placed immediately following surgery as long as it is adequately supported by the abutment teeth and maintains minimal soft tissue contact. In this patient the fixtures were placed in maxillary lateral incisor positions bilaterally, and the provisional restorations were then recemented.

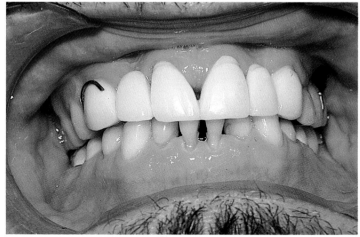

Fig. 5-26

PRELIMINARY IMPRESSIONS

Once adequate time for osseointegration has passed, the implants are exposed and abutment cylinders are placed. Upon healing of the soft tissues, fabrication of the definitive fixed partial denture can begin.

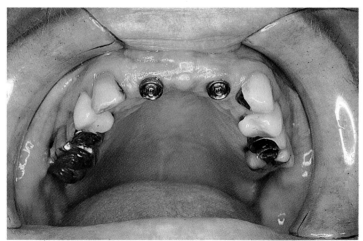

Fig. 5-27

Tapered Impression Copings

Preliminary impressions are made with tapered impression copings. The abutments are cleaned and tightened, and the copings are screwed into place. An irreversible hydrocolloid impression is made with a stock tray.

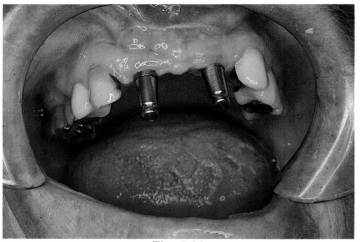

Fig. 5-28

The tapered impression copings remain intraorally when the impression tray is removed.

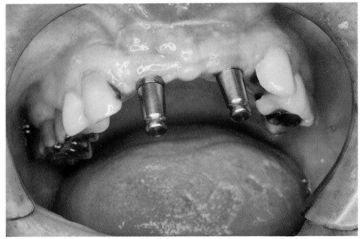

Fig. 5-29

Brass Analogues

The impression copings are removed from the patient, connected to brass analogues, and inserted securely back into the impression.

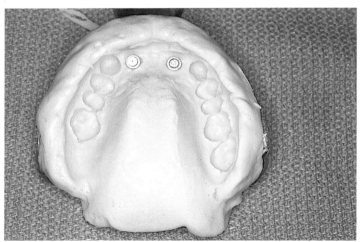

Fig. 5-30

Preliminary Casts

The preliminary impression is poured with improved dental stone. The impression and copings are removed and the preliminary cast is trimmed.

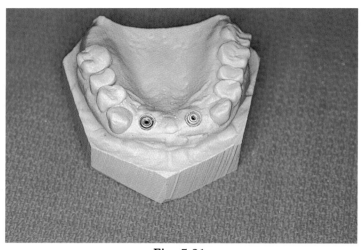

Fig. 5-31

MASTER IMPRESSIONS

Square Impression Copings

Square impression copings, which will be utilized in making the master impression, are placed on the preliminary cast in order to fabricate the master impression tray.

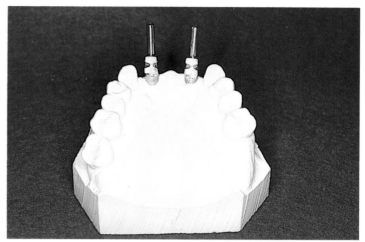

Fig. 5-32

Wax is used to block out undercuts on the cast and impression copings and insure proper thickness of impression material in the desired locations.

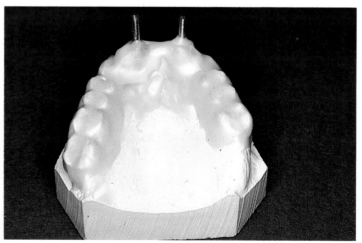

Fig. 5-33

Master Impression Tray

The master impression tray is fabricated so that the long guide screws exit the tray as shown.

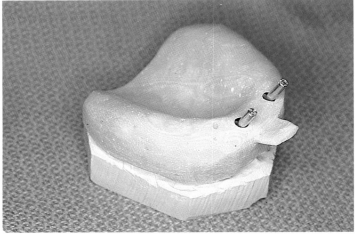

Fig. 5-34

If different abutment lengths are desired, they must be changed prior to making the master impression. The abutments are cleaned and tightened, and the square impression copings are positioned.

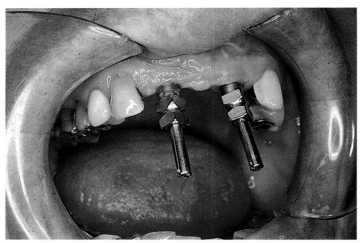

Fig. 5-35

Impression Technique

Impression material is syringed, thoroughly encompassing the copings.

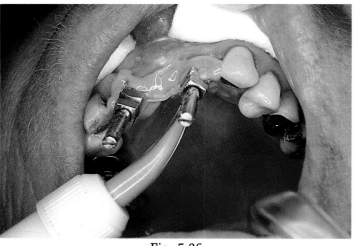

Fig. 5-36

The impression tray, filled with a heavy body impression material, is seated. Once the material has polymerized, the long guide screws are loosened but not removed from the impression.

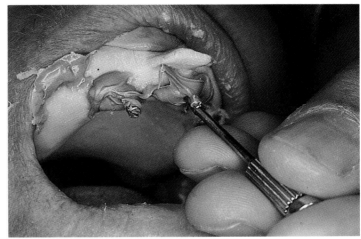

Fig. 5-37

The tray is removed with the square copings and guide screws positioned within the impression material.

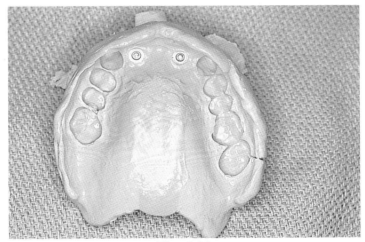

Fig. 5-38

This sectioned impression illustrates how the square copings become locked within the impression material. The tray cannot be removed until the guide screw is loosened, releasing the impression coping from the abutment.

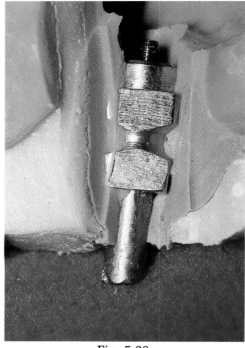

Fig. 5-39

Brass analogues are connected to the impression copings and the master cast is fabricated.

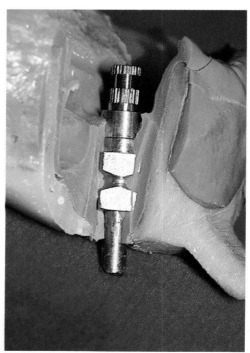

Fig. 5-40

Limited access in the posterior regions makes it difficult to loosen the long guide screws, especially in the presence of opposing dentition. It may be necessary to shorten the guide screws in these situations.

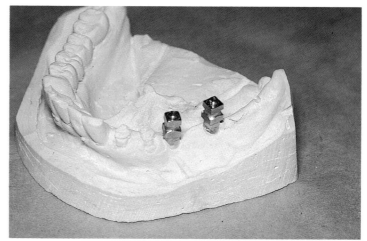

Fig. 5-41

The shortened guide screws must extend through the impression tray.

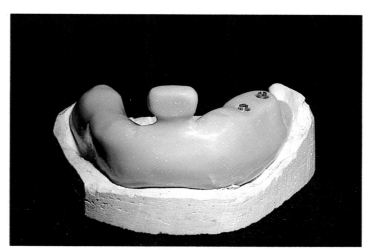

Fig. 5-42

Even with shortened guide screws, access still may be difficult.

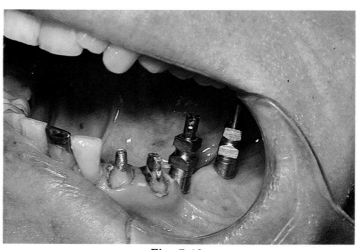

Fig. 5-43

Because of impaired access, it is sometimes necessary to utilize the tapered copings for making master impressions. While their use adds a source of possible error due to the fact that they are removed from and then placed back into the impression, there may be no alternative. Discrepancies can be noted at the time of the metal try-in and can be resolved with a solder relation record.

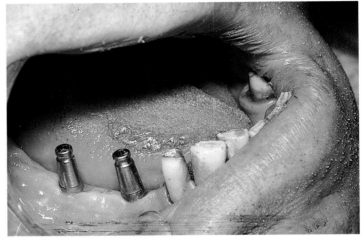

Fig. 5-44

No one particular impression material is preferred. To accurately hold the impression copings in proper position, however, it is best to use a rigid material. But in this patient a light bodied material was utilized due to the large number of natural tooth preparations present and a need for greater working time.

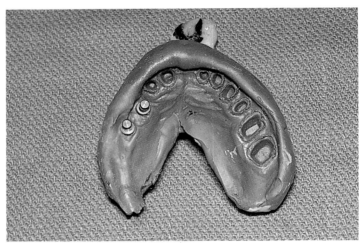

Fig. 5-45

Master Casts

The master casts are fabricated with improved dental stone using recommended liquid/powder ratios (Figs. 5-46,A and B).

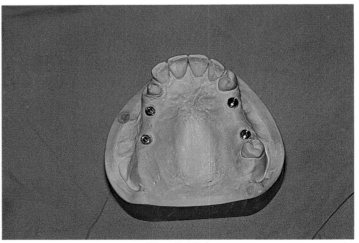

Fig. 5-46,A

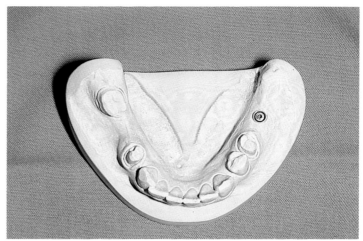

Fig. 5-46,B

REGISTRATIONS

Record bases may be necessary in order to make appropriate maxillo/mandibular records. Gold cylinders are incorporated within the acrylic resin record bases (Figs. 5-47,A and B). Short guide pins or gold screws are used to secure the record intraorally. The records are then made in the usual manner and transferred to an articulator.

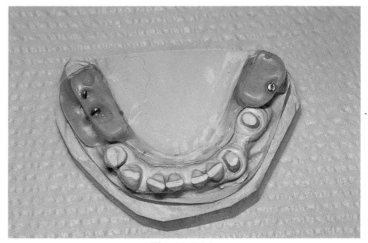

Fig. 5-47,A

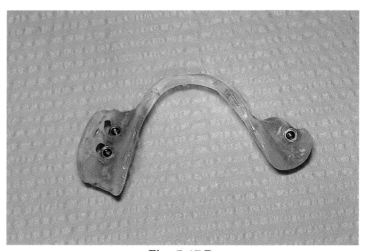

Fig. 5-47,B

The master casts are mounted in preparation for fabrication of the definitive restoration (Figs. 5-48,A and B).

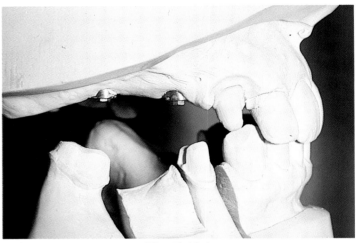

Fig. 5-48,A

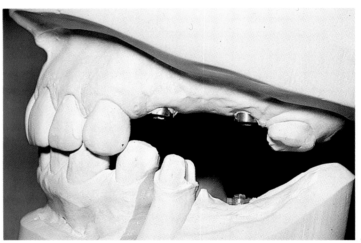

Fig. 5-48,B

PROSTHESIS FABRICATION

Gold Cylinders

The gold cylinders, which will eventually become incorporated into the final restoration, are placed on the brass analogues. These cylinders are available in heights of 3.0 mm and 4.0 mm.

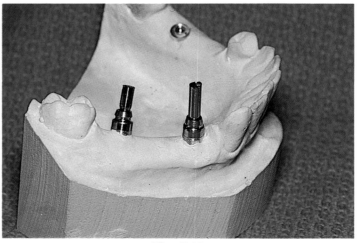

Fig. 5-49

Wax Pattern

The wax pattern of the definitive restoration is prepared incorporating the gold cylinders. The bottom 1.5 to 2 mms of the gold cylinders should be free of wax. This particular wax pattern is designed for a resin-to-metal restoration. Initially, resin was considered the occlusal material of choice for implant-supported fixed partial dentures. However, the high rate of fracture of this material has raised serious doubts as to its applicability for implant-supported restorations.

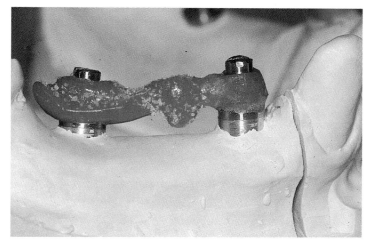

Fig. 5-50

The gold cylinders must be free of wax or debris prior to investing.

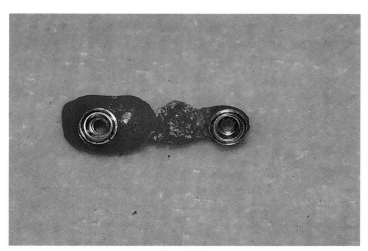

Fig. 5-51

This wax pattern is designed for a porcelain fused to metal restoration. Note that the wax pattern terminates 1.5-2 mm short of the bottom of the gold cylinders (Figs. 5-52,A and B).

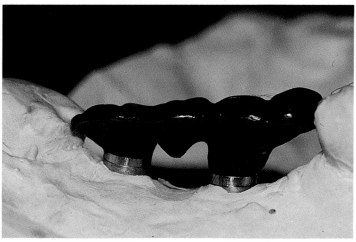

Fig. 5-52,A

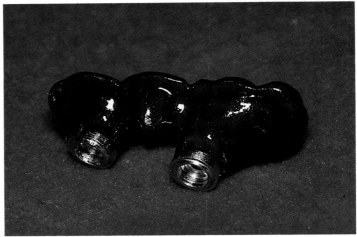

Fig. 5-52,B

Casting

The wax pattern is sprued, invested, and cast.

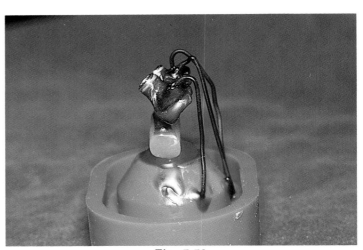

Fig. 5-53

The metal casting is cleaned, and the internal aspects of the gold cylinders are checked under a microscope. The casting is then seated on the working cast.

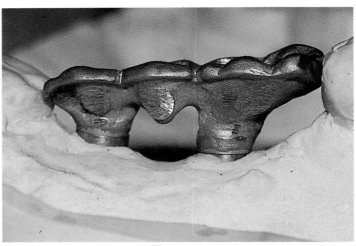

Fig. 5-54

Metal Try-in

The metal casting is seated intraorally prior to completing the restoration. The framework must seat completely and passively. A discrepancy, which is easily discernable with this system, requires a solder relation record.

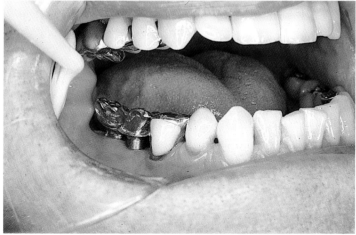

Fig. 5-55

Definitive Restoration

If the final restoration is to be porcelain fused to metal, the porcelain can now be added in a conventional manner. In this patient, the opposing occlusion was porcelain, and so a porcelain occlusal surface was designed.

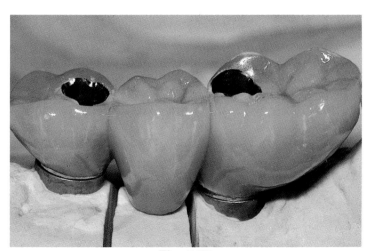

Fig. 5-56

The restoration is ready for placement. The screw access holes initially will be sealed with cotton and temporary cement.

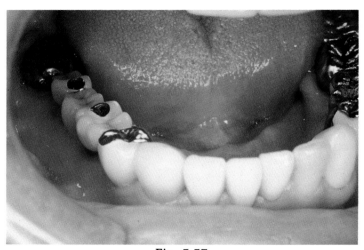

Fig. 5-57

Occlusal Materials

Porcelain has been used extensively by the UCLA group with no obvious detrimental effects. To date, the only complication has been a porcelain fracture affectng one restoration. The clinical followup period, however, is short (1-4 year followup). Long-term clinical studies are necessary to evaluate the true effect of the available occlusal materials on the long-term success of osseointegrated implants (Figs. 5-58,A and B).

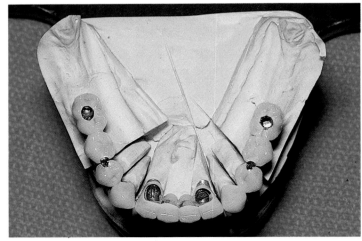

Fig. 5-58,A

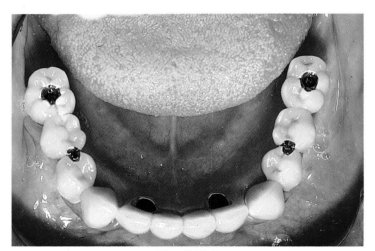

Fig. 5-58,B

The criteria for selecting occlusal materials is currently based on the opposing occlusion. The mandibular arch in this patient (Figs. 5-59,A and B) contained metal occlusal surfaces, and so the implant-supported restorations were fabricated with metal occlusal surfaces.

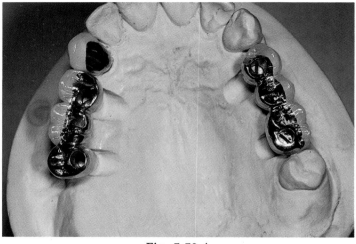

Fig. 5-59,A

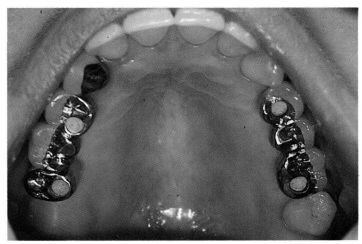

Fig. 5-59,B

No one particular occlusal material is favored in the fabrication of an implant-supported fixed partial denture. This patient was satisfied with the existing gold restoration on the second premolar. The opposing occlusion was natural dentition, and the material of choice for this implant-supported restoration was type III gold alloy.

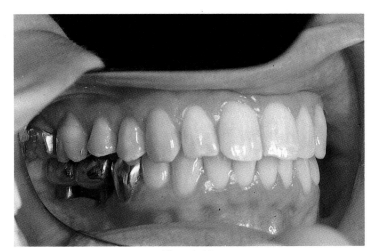

Fig. 5-60

In summary, a consensus has not yet formed with respect to the selection and effects of the occlusal materials available for implant-supported fixed partial dentures. In the authors' experience, it appears that current resins may not be suitable materials becase of their high rate of fracture (Fig. 5-61,A).

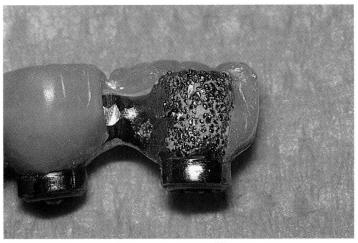

Fig. 5-61,A

Conversely, only one porcelain restoration has fractured to date (Fig. 5-61,B).

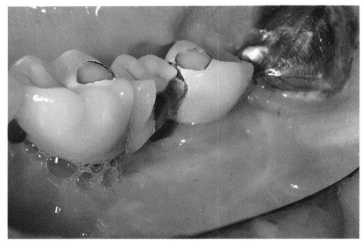

Fig. 5-61,B

The restoration is secured with the gold screws and the screw access holes are filled with gutta percha (Fig. 5-62,A) prior to sealing with resin (Fig. 5-62,B).

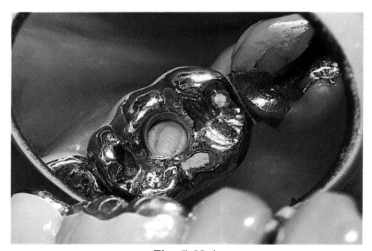

Fig. 5-62,A

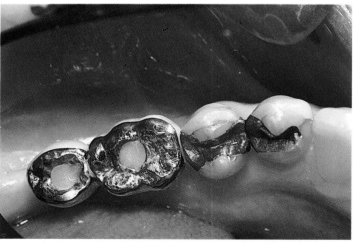

Fig. 5-62,B

Radiographs

Radiographs are made to assure proper seating of the abutment cylinders and the definitive restoration (Figs. 5-63,A and B).

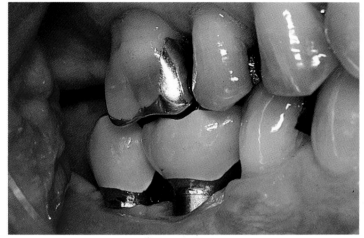

Fig. 5-63,A

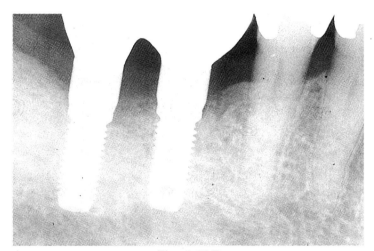

Fig. 5-63,B

Occlusal Consideration

It appears desirable, particularly when implants are considered for the maxilla, that natural dentition provide anterior guidance during lateral excursion. This natural maxillary canine enjoys excellent periodontal support and provides anterior guidance (See Fig. 5-4,A). The posterior restoration maintains occlusal contacts only in centric relation. It is recommended that if adequate anterior guidance with the natural dentition exists, the implant supported restoration be free of excursive contacts.

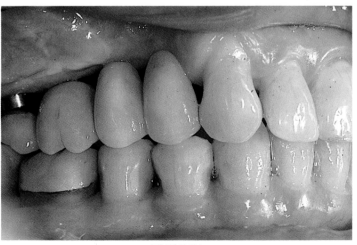

Fig. 5-64

Maxillary teeth posterior to the left lateral incisor were absent in this patient. A panoramic radiograph revealed adequate bone for the placement of two maxillary implants, but the distal-most fixture could be placed no further posteriorly than the second premolar region. The natural dentition did not provide adequate anterior guidance on the left side, and so the implant-supported fixed partial denture made contact in both centric relation and lateral excursion. Rather than use the cantilevered canine for anterior guidance, group function was developed to distribute the lateral forces evenly over the entire restoration.

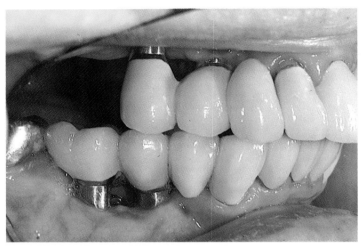

Fig. 5-65

Due to compromised bone density in the maxillary arch, a more conservative approach is taken in the fabrication of implant-supported restorations. The original prosthesis for this patient (see Fig. 5-65) extended no further posteriorly than the distal abutment. One year of initial loading was allowed. The restoration was then removed and a new prosthesis fabricated. The new restoration included a posterior cantilever. It should be remembered that osseointegration continues to improve after the abutments are connected, and therefore more can be asked of an implant once it has been loaded for an extended period of time.[1] It is for this reason that proper treatment of maxillary implants may include minimal initial loading, with progressive increases over time. Implant supported fixed provisional restorations could be useful for this purpose.

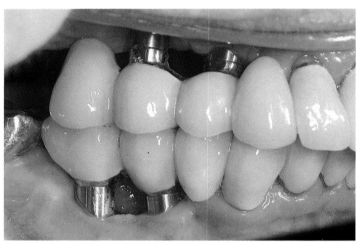

Fig. 5-66

IMPLANT-NATURAL TOOTH RESTORATION

Biologic Differences

The evidence is unclear whether an implant supported restoration should be connected directly to natural dentition. When implants are indicated, it is best to place two or more. In this way the prosthesis can be designed independent of the natural dentition. There are some patients where this is not possible and the restoration must be supported by both natural dentition and an individual implant.

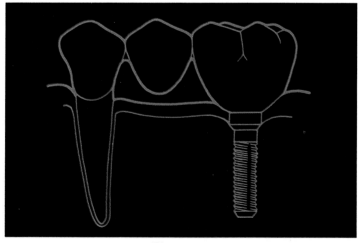

Fig. 5-67

Stress Breaking Attachments

A non-rigid attachment was used in this restoration in order to avoid a direct connection between the natural dentition (first pre-molar and cuspid) and the osseointegrated implant. The efficacy of this method of attachment however requires further study (Figs. 5-68,A and B).

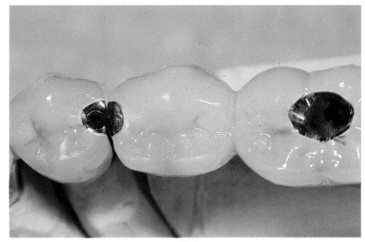

Fig. 5-68,A

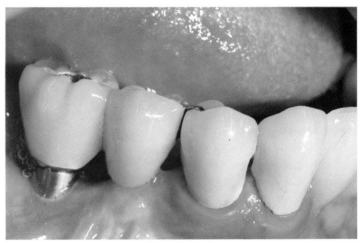

Fig. 5-68,B

An occlusal view of the restorations shown in Figure 5-68,B demonstrates the non-rigid interlock attachment in the distal of the first premolar. The attachment provides vertical and horizontal support and prevents rotation and loosening of the screw retaining the implant supported restoration. An additional advantage gained is the retriev ability of the implant supported portion of the restoration.

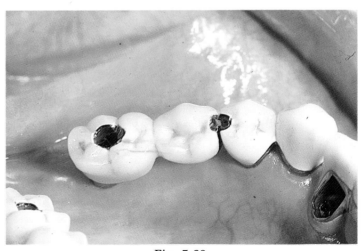

Fig. 5-69

Telescopic Copings

Some clinicians prefer to utilize telescopic copings, as opposed to attachments, for uniting the implant-supported restoration to the natural dentition. The desired means of connection remains unclear and requires further study. It is apparent, however, that retrievability is an important factor in restorations associated with osseointegrated implants (Figs. 5-70,A, B, and C).

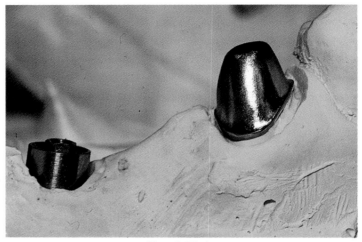

Fig. 5-70,A

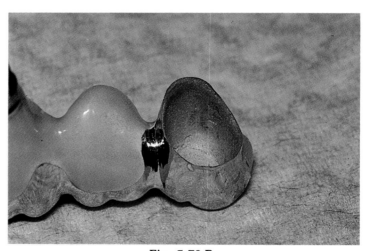

Fig. 5-70,B

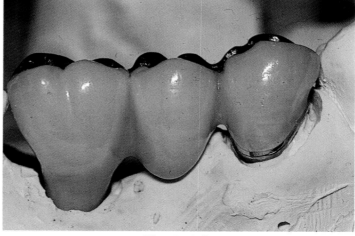

Fig. 5-70,C

UCLA ABUTMENT[2]

The UCLA abutment was developed to allow direct connection between the implant-supported restoration and the top of the implant fixture, eliminating the need for the tansmucosal abutment cylinder.

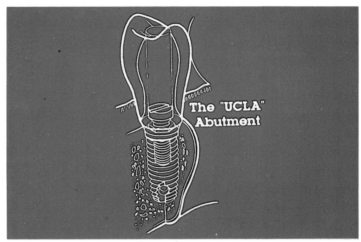

Fig. 5-71

Indications

The anterior edentulous span in this patient was too great to restore with a conventional fixed partial denture. The patient did not wish to be restored with a removable partial denture, so four implants were placed. In this clinical situation, bypassing the transmucosal abutment cylinders and fabricating the restoration directly to the implant fixtures will improve the esthetic result dramatically since porcelain rather than titanium will emerge from the perimplant soft tissues.

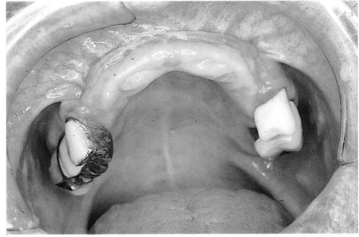

Fig. 5-72

In this patient, besides the obvious esthetic considerations, insufficient interocclusal space exists for the fabrication of the implant-supported restoration using the conventional components.

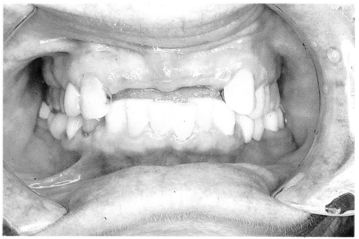

Fig. 5-73

The mounted diagnostic casts reveal limited interocclusal working space. Gold cylinders cannot be placed in this situation.

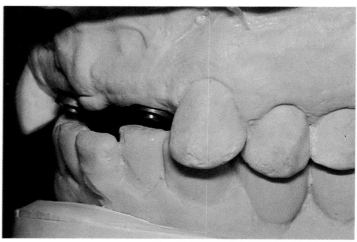

Fig. 5-74

Design Considerations

The UCLA abutment is a machined plastic pattern designed to engage the implant fixture. This plastic component becomes incorporated within the wax pattern. The resulting casting will therefore fit precisely atop the implant fixture.

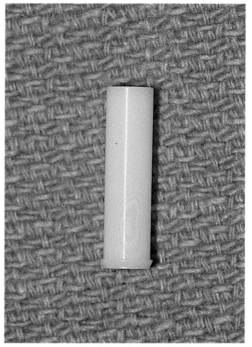

Fig. 5-75

Illustrated is the UCLA abutment connected to the implant fixture. The base of the pattern contains a collar. This collar can be increased in size by adding wax, or it can be left as is. Once cast, the metal collar provides structural support for the base of the restoration.

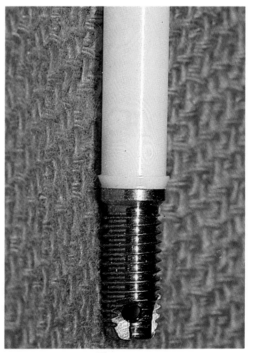

Fig. 5-76

The slight vertical extension at the base of the abutment allows for milling of the restoration once it is cast. The milling process ensures close adaptation between the cast restoration and the implant fixture.

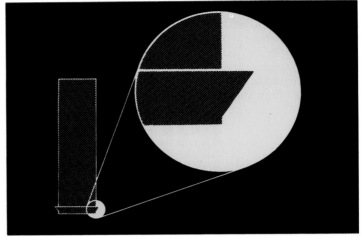

Fig. 5-77

In summary, using the conventional components, the dental restoration is designed to engage the transmucosal abutment cylinders (Fig. 5-78,A).

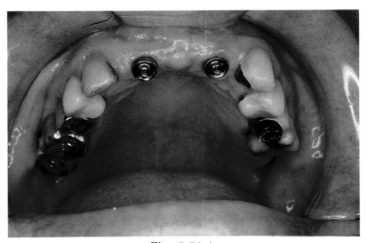

Fig. 5-78,A

The working cast with the brass abutment analogues is shown in Figure 5-78,B.

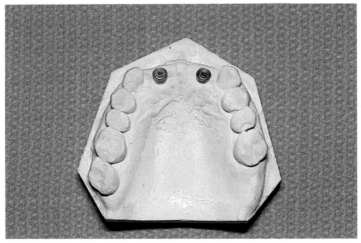

Fig. 5-78,B

With the "UCLA" abutment, the restoration is designed to engage the implant fixtures (Fig. 5-78,C).

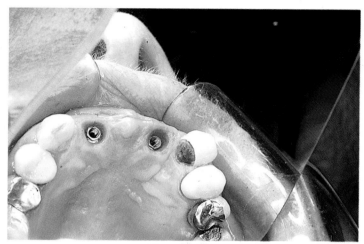

Fig. 5-78,C

The working cast with implant fixture analogues embedded is shown in Figure 5-78,D.

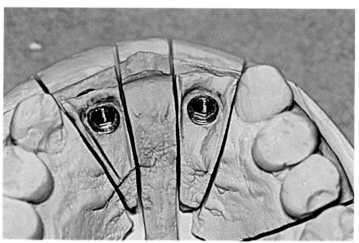

Fig. 5-78,D

Master Impressions

Preliminary impressions are made in the conventional manner using tapered impression copings. A master impression tray is fabricated on the preliminary cast. The square impression copings are used for the master impression.

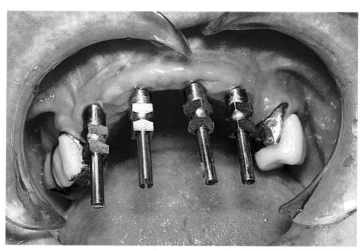

Fig. 5-79

Impression material is syringed around the impression copings. The tray is filled and seated.

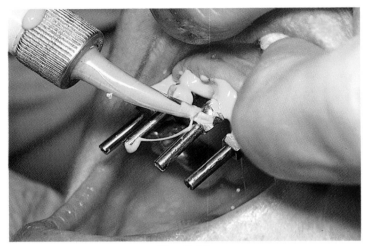

Fig. 5-80

The guide screws are loosened and the impression is removed. The bottom of guide screws and copings can be seen in the impression.

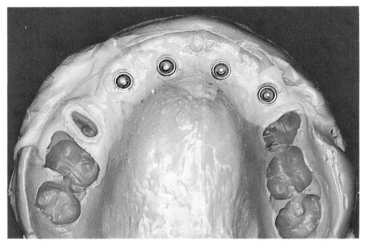

Fig. 5-81

With the conventional method, the brass analogues are connected to the impression copings. With the "UCLA" abutment technique, a fixture analogue and an abutment analogue are connected to each impression coping.

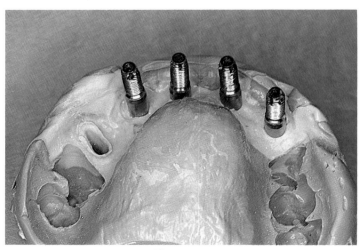

Fig. 5-82

In Figure 5-83,A the brass analogue has been connected to the impression coping, whereas in Figure 5-83,B when utilizing the "UCLA" abutment technique, a fixture analogue and abutment analogue are attached to the impression coping. The size of the abutment analogue used in the impression must be identical to that used in the patient to ensure that the fixture analogue is embedded in the master cast at the proper subgingival level.

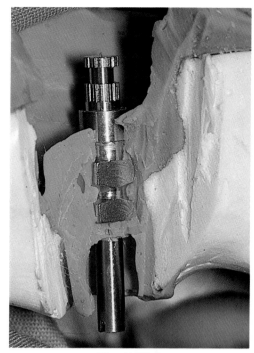

Fig. 5-83,A

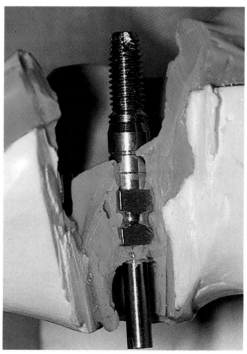

Fig. 5-83,B

Wax is applied to the surface of the abutment cylinder as shown. This allows for easy retrieval of the abutment cylinder from the master cast.

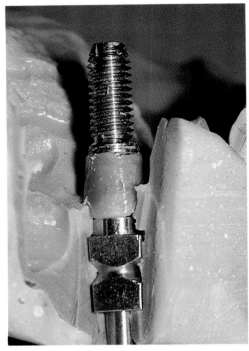

Fig. 5-84

Master Cast

The impression is poured in improved dental stone and the tray removed. The master cast contains fixture and abutment analogues.

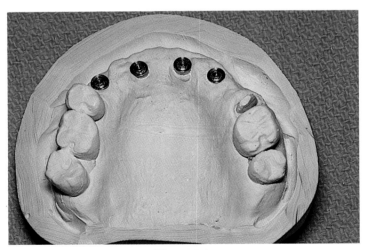

Fig. 5-85

Stone is relieved from the lingual side in some instances, to remove the abutment analogues from the master cast. The stone representing the buccal gingival contours must be retained when fabricating anterior restorations.

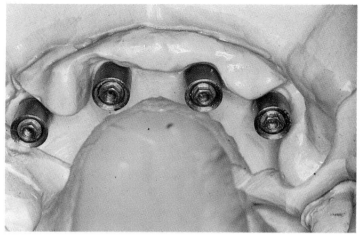

Fig. 5-86

The abutment cylinder analogues are removed, exposing the fixture analogues.

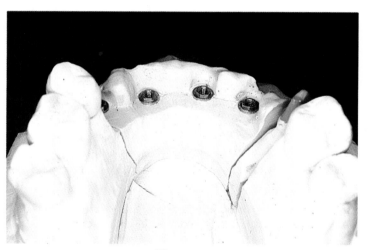

Fig. 5-87

Wax Pattern

The plastic "UCLA" abutment is placed on the fixture analogue and sectioned at the appropriate occlusal level. The entire screw access channel should be cast in metal to provide for proper support of the porcelain.

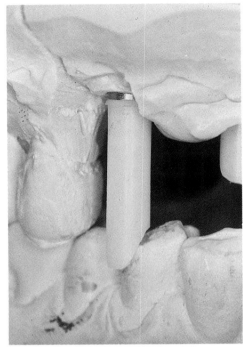

Fig. 5-88

Wax is added to the abutment in order to develop the wax pattern. The design is determined by the choice of the final restoration. The design of this restoration will allow porcelain to cover the entire buccal surface except for a small metal collar at the base.

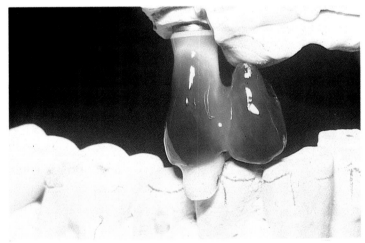

Fig. 5-89

Wax patterns are developed in individual segments, one for each implant fixture.

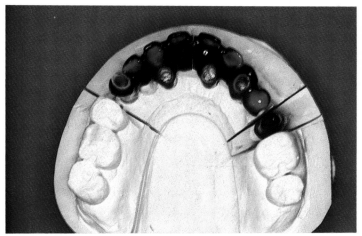

Fig. 5-90

The lingual surface will be in metal.

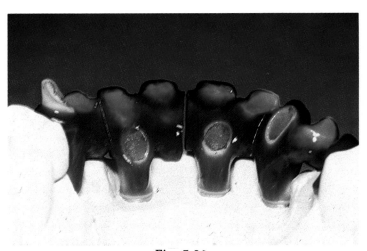

Fig. 5-91

This section is ready to be invested and cast. The plastic pattern will be eliminated with the wax. Care must be taken in the development of subgingival contours and the emergence profile so as to promote a healthy gingival response and facilitate oral hygiene access.

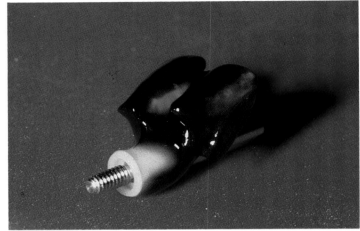

Fig. 5-92

Metal Framework

The metal castings are seated on the master cast.

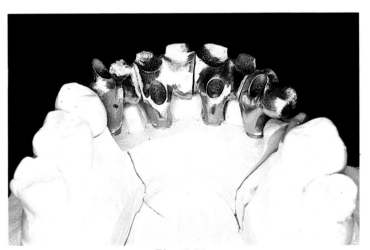

Fig. 5-93

The milling device (Fig. 5-94,A) is used with the abrasive paste to refine the undersurface of the restoration (Fig. 5-94,B).

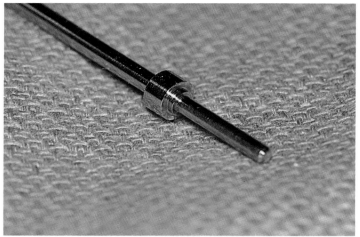

Fig. 5-94,A

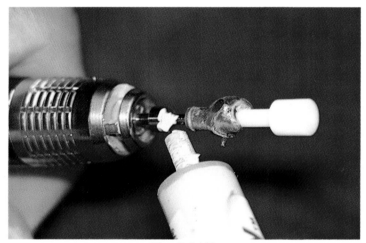

Fig. 5-94,B

The adaptation of the milled casting to the implant fixture (Fig. 5-95,A) has been shown microscopically (Fig. 5-95,B) to consistently equal or surpass the adaptation of the conventional components.

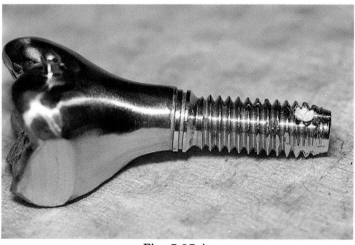

Fig. 5-95,A

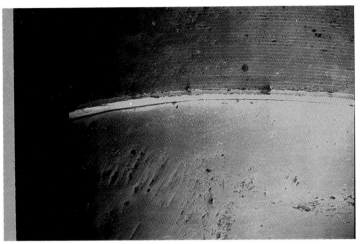

Fig. 5-95,B

The castings are now ready for verification orally.

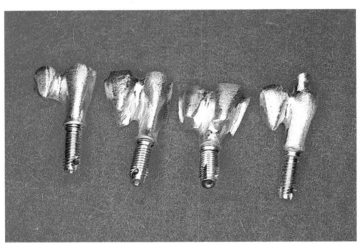

Fig. 5-96

The transmucosal abutment cylinders are removed in preparation for the metal try-in.

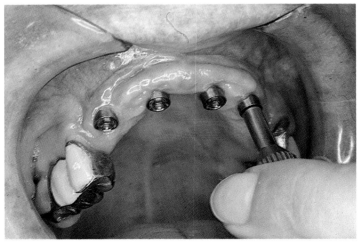

Fig. 5-97

The implant fixtures are exposed and soft tissue tags, which may interfere with seating of castings, are removed.

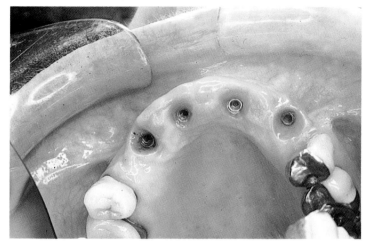

Fig. 5-98

Solder Index

The framework segments are positioned and secured with the titanium screws. It is difficult to detect seating discrepancies at the level of the osseous crest; it is for this reason that the segments are seated individually. Adequate space for solder joints must exist between the segments.

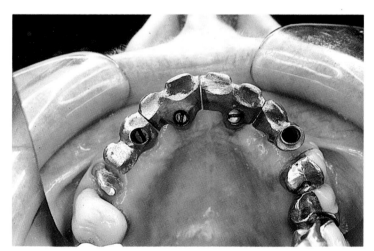

Fig. 5-99

A solder transfer record is made, and the metal framework is removed. It is recommended that the implant analogues be attached to the framework and embedded in a new working cast prior to soldering (Fig. 5-100,A). This new cast will contain the fixtures embedded in their proper position.

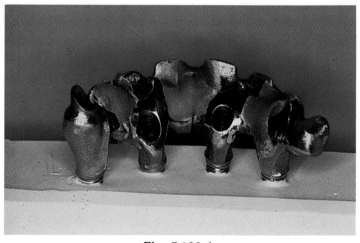

Fig. 5-100,A

Once soldered, the restoration can be placed back onto this cast and the soldered framework can be checked visually to verify the precise fit necessary in these restorations (Fig. 5-100,B).

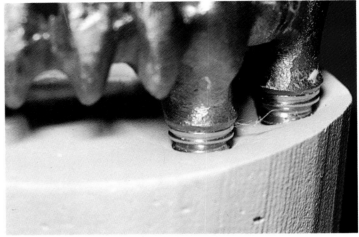

Fig. 5-100,B

Final Restorations

Porcelain is added to the metal framework and the restoration is completed.

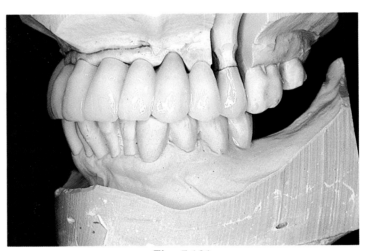

Fig. 5-101

This restoration is designed to extend the porcelain sub-gingivally. A ridge lap design is used in the anterior region when necessary.

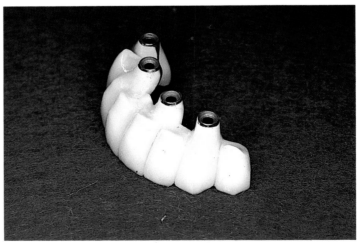

Fig. 5-102

This view shows the design of the lingual screw access holes. The design of the metal framework prevents the fracture of porcelain around the screw access openings.

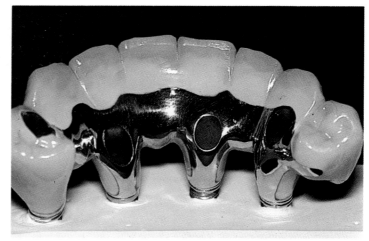

Fig. 5-103

A close-up buccal view illustrates the base of the restoration. The facial porcelain allows for an esthetic gingival emergence of the restoration. Note the metal collar at the base.

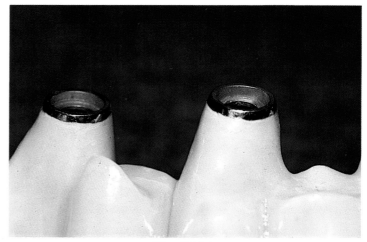

Fig. 5-104

The abutment cylinders are removed and the definitive prosthesis is delivered.

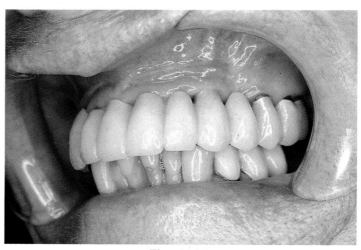

Fig. 5-105

A close-up view of the finished restoration is shown. Note that the canine connects directly to an implant fixture. When initially placed, the soft tissue adjacent to the restoration may blanch. This may indicate the need for recontouring the restoration. Prolonged discomfort and blanching is an indication of tissue entrapment. It is important to avoid entrapment of soft tissue between the restoration and the implant fixture.

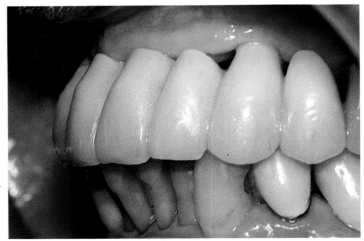

Fig. 5-106

A radiograph is taken to evaluate the junction of the restoration and the implant fixtures.

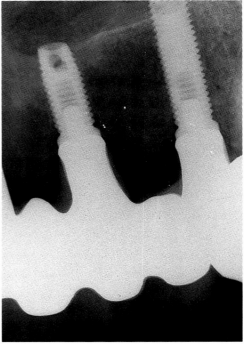

Fig. 5-107

The finished prosthesis provides esthetics similar to that achieved with a conventional tooth-supported porcelain fused to metal restoration.

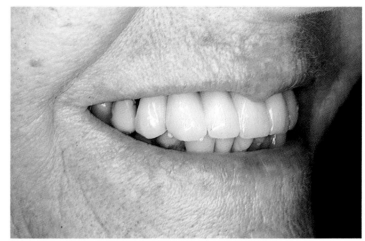

Fig. 5-108

Gingival Response

Note the gingival response upon removal of the restoration six months following delivery.

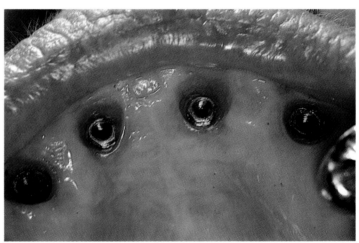

Fig. 5-109

Illustrated is an implant-supported fixed partial denture with the posterior unit fabricated in a conventional manner and the anterior unit fabricated with the UCLA abutment. The tissue response around both the titanium and porcelain abutments is excellent. It appears that there is less plaque accumulation in this patient on the highly glazed porcelain surface fabricated with the "UCLA" abutment than on the surface of the machined titanium abutment cylinder.

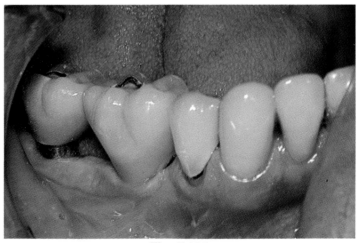

Fig. 5-110

Note the emergence profiles of these implant-supported restorations fabricated with the "UCLA" abutment (Figs. 5-111,A and B). By beginning the contours of the restoration at the implant fixture, more natural emergence profiles can be developed.

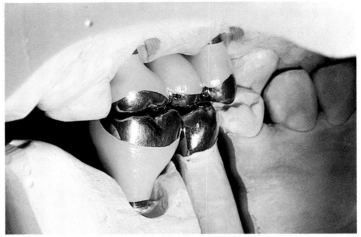

Fig. 5-111,A

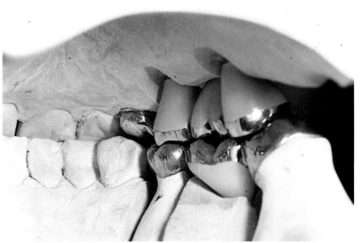

Fig. 5-111,B

Note the completed restoration (Figs. 5-112,A and B). A pleasing esthetic appearance has been achieved without compromising oral hygiene access.

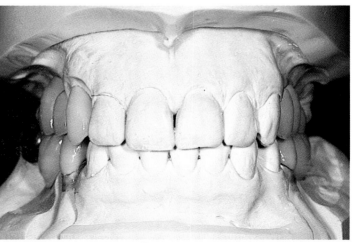

Fig. 5-112,A

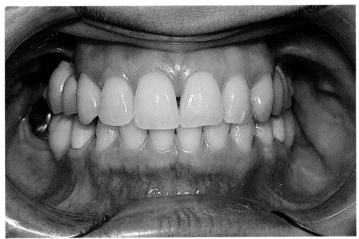

Fig. 5-112,B

Emergence profiles as seen from the labial (Figs. 5-113,A and B) and palatal (Figs 5-113,C and D) promote good oral hygiene and a healthy soft tissue response. Appropriate position and angulation of implant fixtures is necessary to achieve the ideal contours shown.

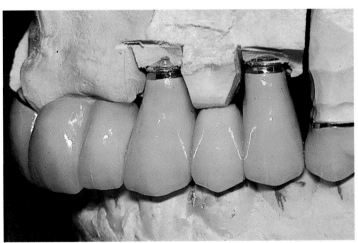

Fig. 5-113,A

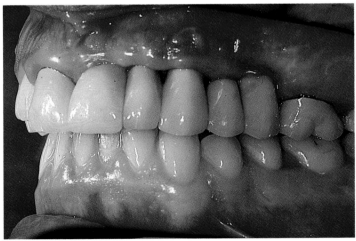

Fig. 5-113,B

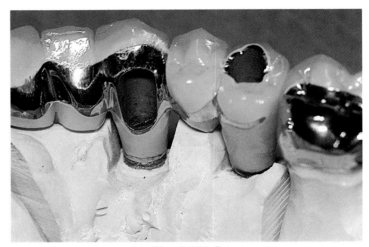

Fig. 5-113,C

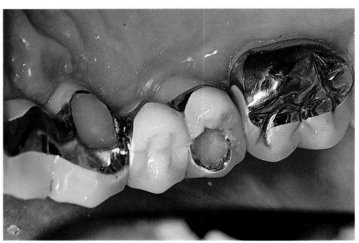

Fig. 5-113,D

Limited Interocclusal Space

In this patient limited interocclusal space is evident clinically and on the mounted diagnostic casts. Fabrication of an implant-supported restoration using the conventional components is not possible (Figs. 5-114,A and B).

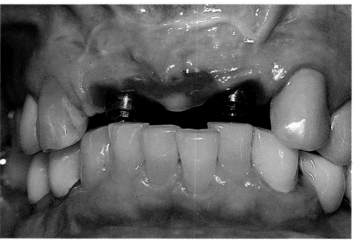

Fig. 5-114,A

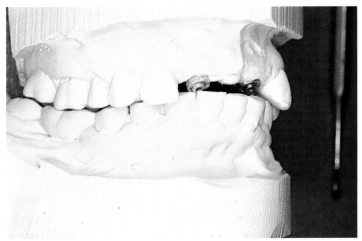

Fig. 5-114,B

The mounted master casts with the abutment cylinder analogues removed (Figs. 5-115,A and B) reveal adequate interocclusal space for development of a restoration with ideal contours (Fig. 5-115,C) when using the "UCLA" abutment.

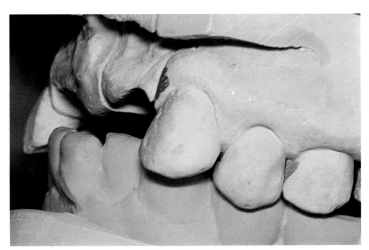

Fig. 5-115,A

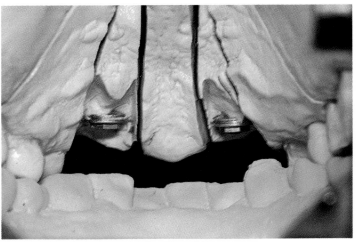

Fig. 5-115,B

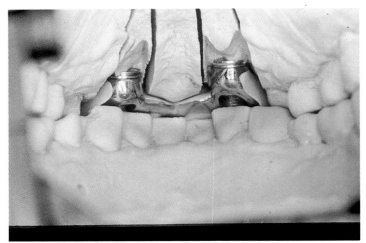

Fig. 5-115,C

The abutment cylinders are removed and the prosthesis is delivered, providing the patient with an extremely favorable esthetic and functional restoration (Figs. 5-116,A, B, and C).

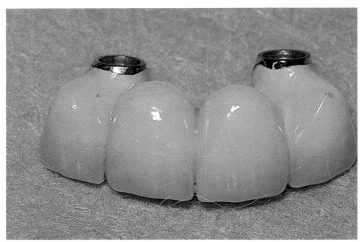

Fig. 5-116,A

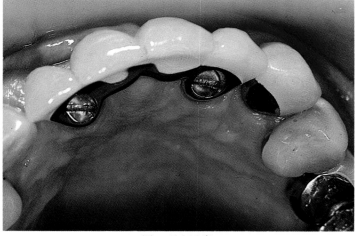

Fig. 5-116,B

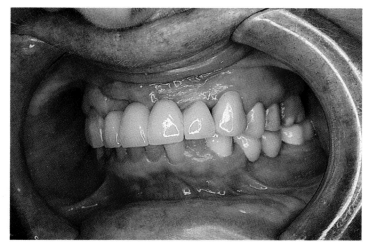

Fig. 5-116,C

Radiographs confirm proper seating of the restoration. Note the direct connection of the restoration to the implant fixture.

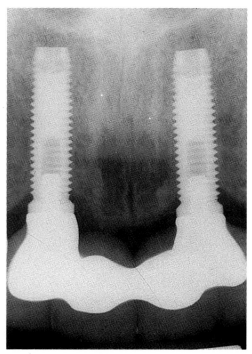

Fig. 5-117

Discrepancies In Angulation

Two mandibular implants were placed anteriorly with excessive buccal inclination. By utilizing the "UCLA" abutment and designing the restoration to attach directly to the implant fixture, the screw access holes can be elongated and the incisal edges of the restoration can be ideally positioned.

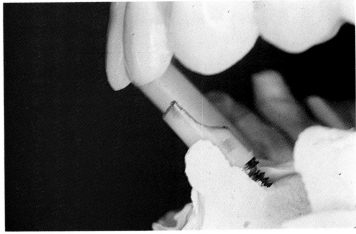

Fig. 5-118

The elongated screw access holes in the completed restoration allows for insertion of screws, enabling development of ideal labial and incisal contours.

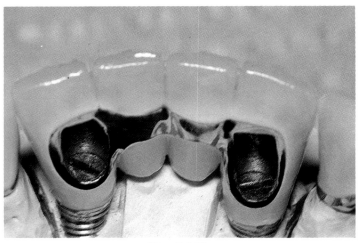

Fig. 5-119

The prosthesis has been inserted. It is apparent that the elongated screw access holes have enabled the development of ideal labial and lingual contours (Figs. 5-120,A and B).

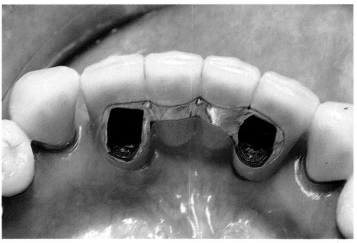

Fig. 5-120,A

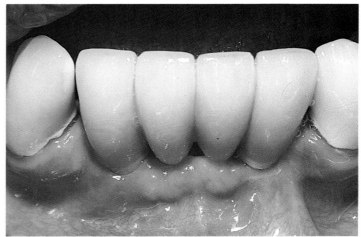

Fig. 5-120,B

Improper angulation of these implant fixtures makes it difficult to fabricate an appropriate prosthesis. The use of surgical stents will usually prevent this occurrence.

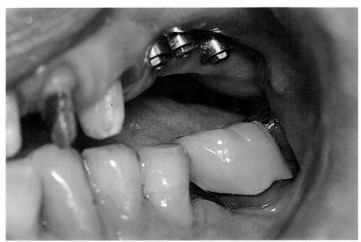

Fig. 5-121

The buccal angulation of the maxillary posterior fixtures is illustrated on this cast.

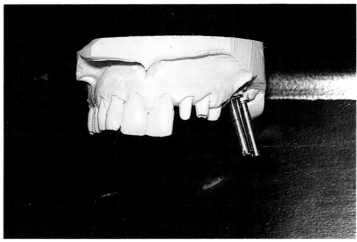

Fig. 5-122

Diagnostic wax-ups or the fabrication of implant supported provisional restorations will reveal problems which might not be evident due to the angle of the implant fixtures. In this patient, the posterior screw access hole was acceptable as it emerged through the occlusal portion of the restoration. The two anterior fixtures were angled to the buccal and the screw access holes would emerge improperly through the facial aspect of the restoration.

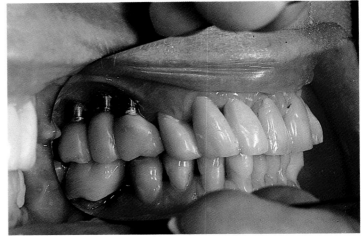

Fig. 5-123

Mounted master casts were prepared for fabrication of the prosthesis. It was planned to fabricate telescopic copings directly to the two anterior implant fixtures utilizing the UCLA abutment.

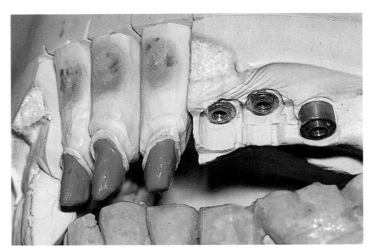

Fig. 5-124

The telescopic copings contained the screw access openings on the facial. Parallel retentive grooves were placed to compensate for the loss of retention due to the presence of these large openings. The copings were designed as single tooth implant restorations, for they engaged the hexagon atop the implant fixture. This practice is necessary so that the copings are positioned in the mouth in precisely the same fashion as they were on the master cast, otherwise the overcasting will not seat properly (Figs. 5-125,A and B).

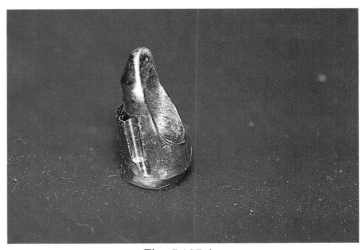

Fig. 5-125,A

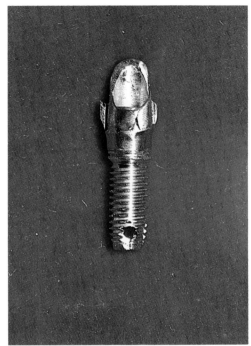

Fig. 5-125,B

The telescopic copings are seated on the master cast. The posterior implant unit will be restored in the conventional fashion.

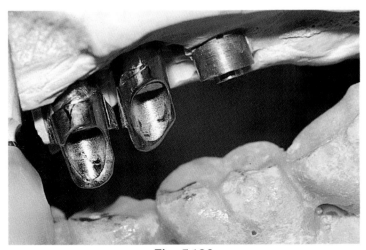

Fig. 5-126

The overcasting is designed and cast. This photograph illustrates the overcasting seated on the telescopic coping, which in turn is secured to an implant fixture.

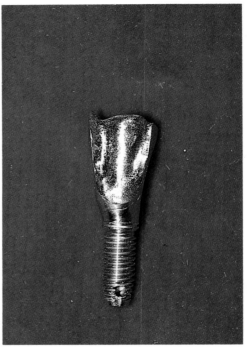

Fig. 5-127

The castings for the porcelain fused to metal restoration are fabricated individually. Two overcastings and one conventional casting are ready for clinical try-in.

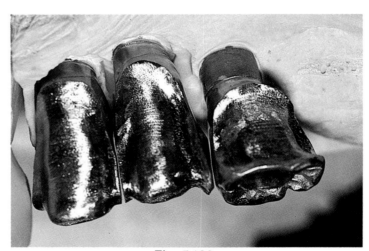

Fig. 5-128

The telescopic copings are secured into position on the two anterior fixtures. The posterior unit is made of the conventional components and is placed on the transmucosal abutment cylinder.

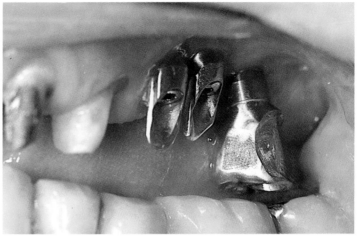

Fig. 5-129

Radiographs are useful to evaluate proper seating of the telescopic copings.

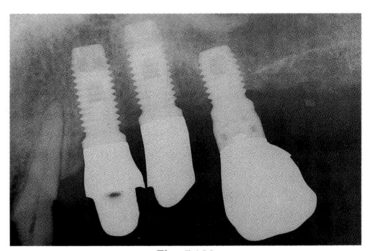

Fig. 5-130

The overcastings are verified intraorally and a solder index is made. Once the three segments are soldered, another try-in of the three-unit metal casting is performed.

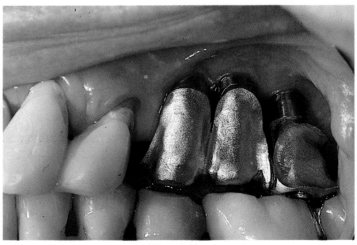

Fig. 5-131

Porcelain is applied and the restoration is completed.

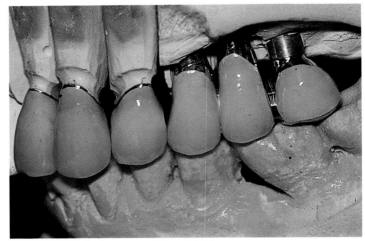

Fig. 5-132

The restoration is positioned by sliding the two anterior over-castings onto the telescopic copings. Posteriorly, the gold cylinder within the molar will provide the connection onto the transmucosal abutment cylinder.

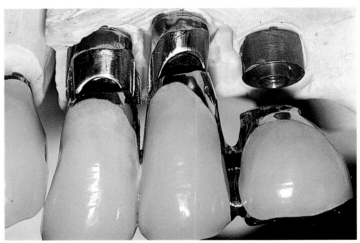

Fig. 5-133

Illustrated is a representation demonstrating the final restoration as connected to the implant fixtures. Only the posterior fixture contains a transmucosal abutment cylinder.

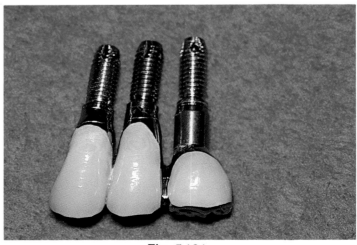

Fig. 5-134

The definitive restoration is in position. Gutta percha is placed over the telescopic coping screws and temporary cement is used to retain the two overcastings. The gold alloy screw in the posterior tooth also retains the restoration. In this way the restoration is retrievable. This utilization of telescopic copings allows the fabrication of a definitive restoration on buccally angled implant fixtures without the contours of the restoration being adversely effected.

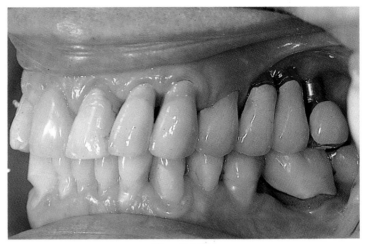

Fig. 5-135

Single-tooth Restorations

Fabrication of single-tooth implant-supported restorations has been difficult. These restorations have had a tendancy to rotate and loosen when occlusal loads are applied, and it has been difficult to achieve acceptable esthetic results using the conventional implant components.

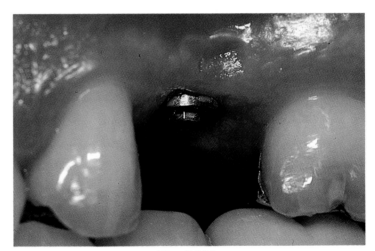

Fig. 5-136

The base of the gold cylinder (Fig. 5-137,A), which becomes part of the final restoration and provides the connection to the abutment, is cylindrical. Therefore, even though it may be tightly screwed in place, it can rotate when subjected to occlusal loads.

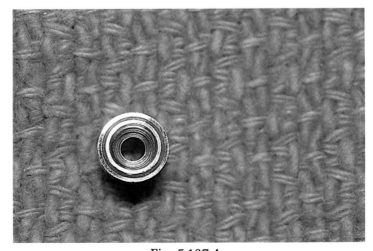

Fig. 5-137,A

The abutment cylinder, however, (Fig. 5-137,B) has a hexagonal shape which matches the hexagon atop the implant fixture. The abutment cylinder cannot freely rotate when properly secured to the implant fixture.

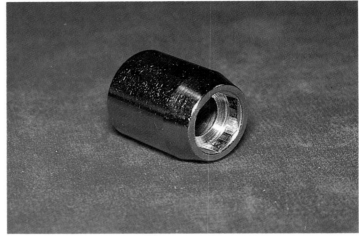

Fig. 5-137,B

Note the hexagon atop the implant fixture.

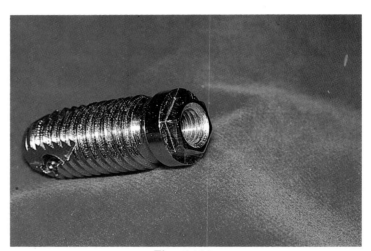

Fig. 5-138

Special single tooth "UCLA" abutments (left) are provided with an internal hexagon at the base to match the hexagon atop the implant fixture. The conventional "UCLA" abutment (right) does not contain the hexagon and is designed for multiple implant-supported fixed partial dentures.

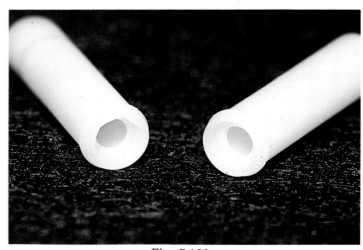

Fig. 5-139

It is critical that the hexagon imbedded within the master cast be in the same rotational alignment as the implant fixture in the patient. To reproduce this alignment, a single tooth impression coping has been designed to fit directly to the implant fixture, engaging the implant fixture hexagon (Figs. 5-140,A and B).

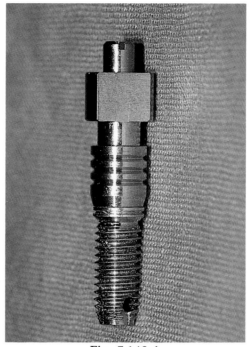

Fig. 5-140,A

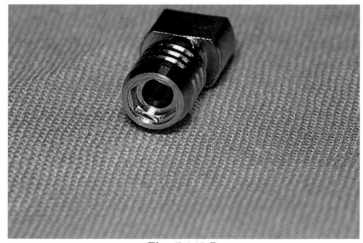

Fig. 5-140,B

A preliminary impression first must be made using a tapered impression coping. The coping, a transmucosal abutment cylinder, and an implant fixture analogue are then positioned back in the impression, and the preliminary cast is poured (Figs. 5-141,A and B).

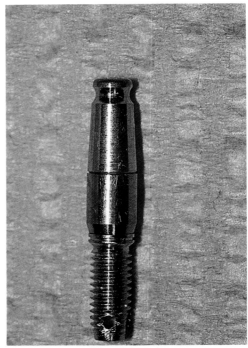

Fig. 5-141,A

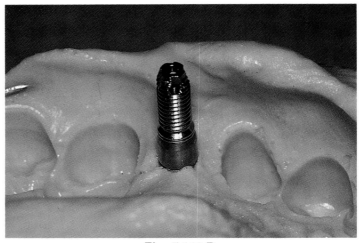

Fig. 5-141,B

The preliminary cast contains an implant fixture analogue in the correct position, but the hexagon on the superior surface is not necessarily in the correct rotational alignment and therefore cannot be used to fabricate the definitive restoration.

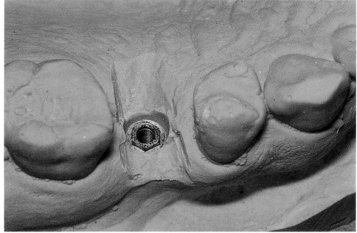

Fig. 5-142

The single-tooth square impression coping is secured to the implant fixture embedded within the preliminary cast.

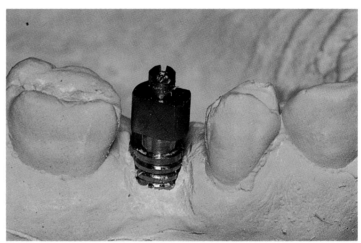

Fig. 5-143

A custom impression tray, which provides access to the long guide pin, is fabricated and will be used for the master impression.

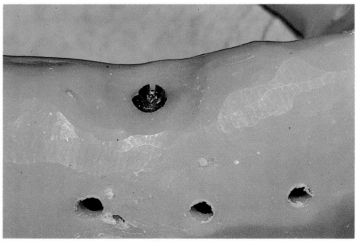

Fig. 5-144

The abutment cylinder is removed and the impression coping placed. If the hexagons are not properly aligned, the impression coping will not seat properly.

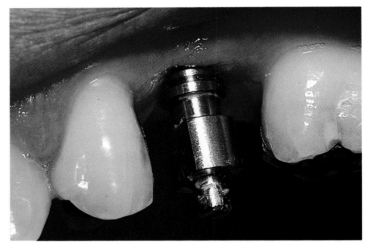

Fig. 5-145

Radiographs can be made to ensure proper seating of the impression coping onto the implant fixture.

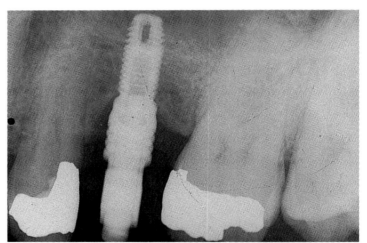

Fig. 5-146

The impression coping remains in the impression material when the tray is removed (Fig. 5-147,A). An implant fixture analogue is connected to the impression coping and the master cast is poured.

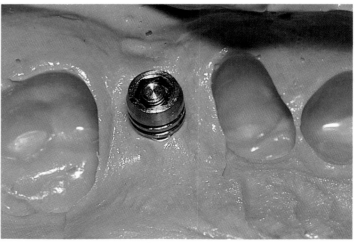

Fig. 5-147,A

A thin layer of wax may be added around the subgingival portion of the impression coping to enhance retrieval of the coping from the stone cast (Fig. 5-147,B).

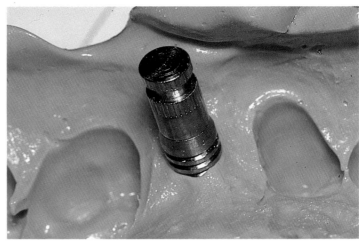

Fig. 5-147,B

The master cast contains the implant fixture analogue (Fig. 5-148,A) with the hexagon in the same rotational alignment as in the patient (Fig. 5-148,B).

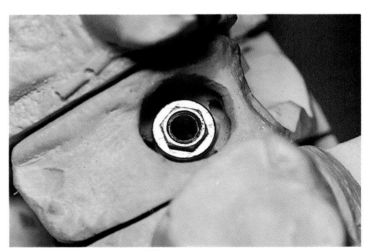

Fig. 5-148,A

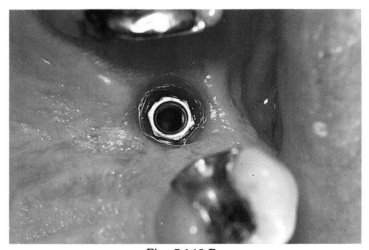

Fig. 5-148,B

The definitive restoration designed with the single-tooth "UCLA" abutment connects to the implant fixture (Figs. 5-149,A and B).

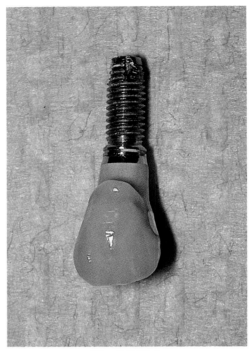

Fig. 5-149,A

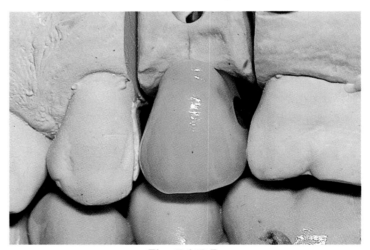

Fig. 5-149,B

The hexagon at the base of this porcelain-fused-to-metal restoration is clearly seen. This design, similar to the transmucosal abutment cylinder, prevents rotation and loosening.

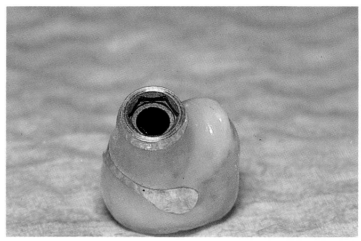

Fig. 5-150

The restoration is placed intraorally.

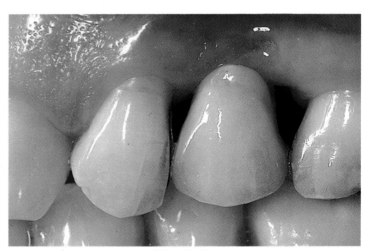

Fig. 5-151

Proper seating of the restoration can be verified with radiographs.

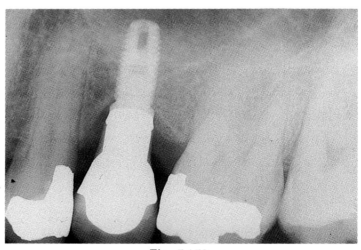

Fig. 5-152

There was sufficient bone available to allow ideal placement of an implant fixture in this patient. Only a minimal ridge-lap (Fig. 5-153,A) was necessary and the lingual contours were ideal (Fig. 5-153,B).

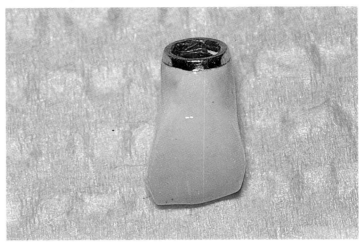

Fig. 5-153,A

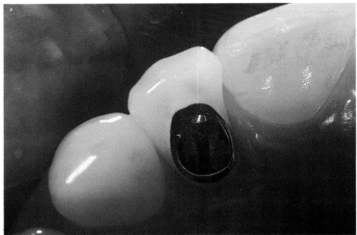

Fig. 5-153,B

This implant-supported lateral incisor provided an excellent esthetic result for this young patient. The highly glazed porcelain discourages plaque retention and promotes a good tissue response. Figure 5-154 represents a two year followup. The restoration had not loosened during the 2 year period.

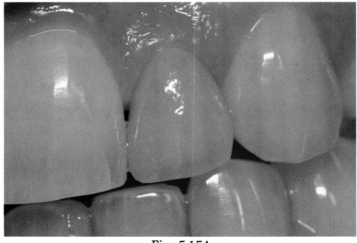

Fig. 5-154

Excessive labial bone resorption followed the loss of this maxillary central incisor, and so the implant fixture was placed palatally Fig. 5-155,A).

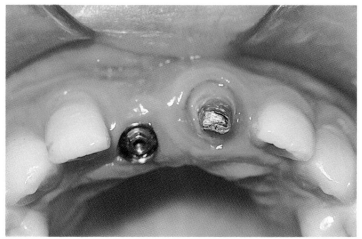

Fig. 5-155,A

In order to achieve an acceptable esthetic result, the implant-supported restoration was ridge lapped (Fig. 5-155,B). The ridge lap design is acceptable in those patients who demonstrate a reasonable level of dental compliance.

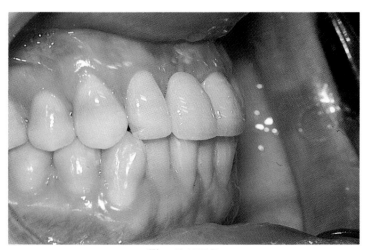

Fig. 5-155,B

NOBELPHARMA SINGLE-TOOTH ABUTMENT

Another method of fabricating single-tooth implant supported restorations utilizes the ''Nobelpharma'' single tooth abutment. These titanium abutment cylinders connect to the implant fixtures, as do conventional transmucosal abutment cylinders. They come in various sizes, depending upon the thickness of the peri-implant tissues (1-5 mm). Restorations are designed to be cemented onto these abutments. The resulting two piece element (crown and abutment cylinder) is then connected to the implant fixture with a titanium screw.

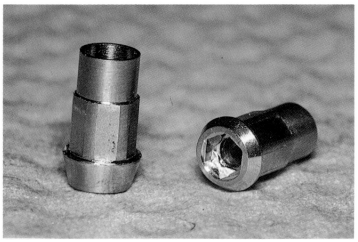

Fig. 5-156

A master cast is fabricated incorporating an implant fixture analgoue. By using a single tooth impression coping, the rotational alignment of the implant hexagon should be correct.

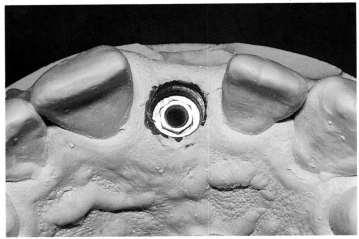

Fig. 5-157

The single-tooth abutment cylinder is secured to the implant fixture (Fig. 5-158,A) and sectioned at the appropriate level (Fig. 5-158,B) so as to allow the fabrication of the single crown over it.

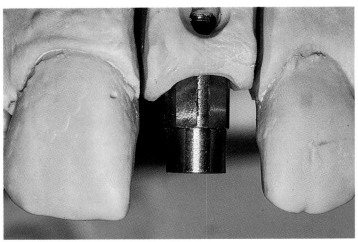

Fig. 5-158,A

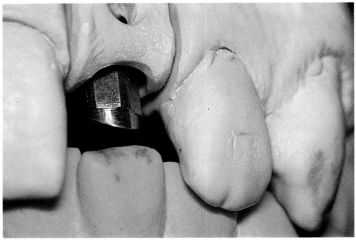

Fig. 5-158,B

The single-tooth abutment connects directly to the implant fixture. By knowing the sulcular depth (measured with the single-tooth impression coping), an appropriate size abutment may be selected. Illustrated is the collar on the abutment cylinder which provides a titanium-soft tissue junction subgingivally yet still allows a slightly subgingival porcelain margin for improved esthetics.

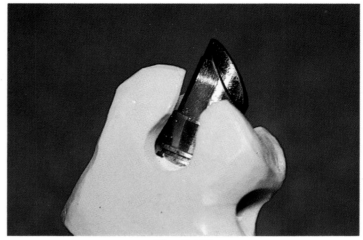

Fig. 5-159

The wax pattern is fabricated on the single-tooth abutment (Figs. 5-160,A and B) and cast in a type V gold alloy.

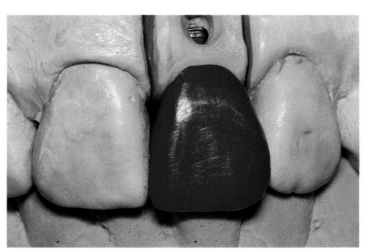

Fig. 5-160,A

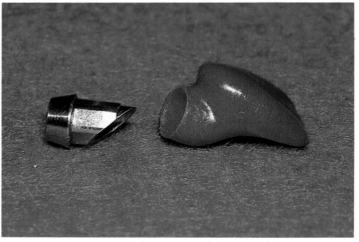

Fig. 5-160,B

The single-tooth casting fits precisely over the single tooth abutment cylinder (Figs. 5-161,A and B).

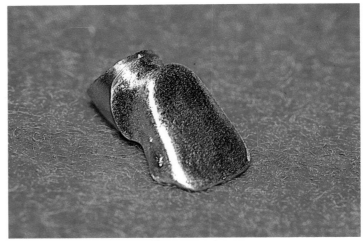

Fig. 5-161,A

Figure 5-161,B illustrates the casting on the abutment cylinder, which in turn is connected to an implant fixture.

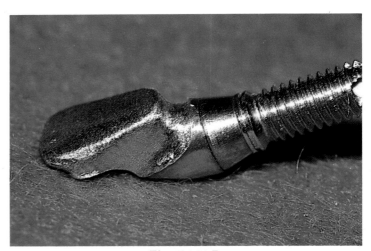

Fig. 5-161,B

The casting is ready for the application of porcelain. Note the subgingival titanium collar of the abutment cylinder (Figs. 5-162,A and B).

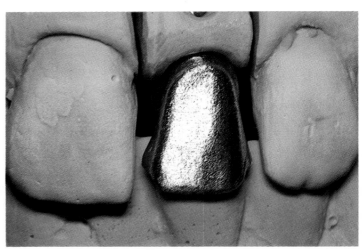

Fig. 5-162,A

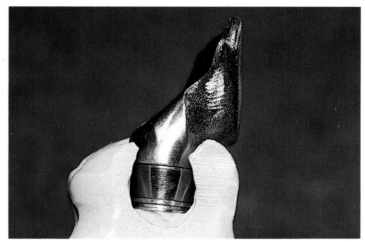

Fig. 5-162,B

Porcelain is applied, and the single-tooth restoration is ready to be evaluated clinically (Fig. 5-163,A).

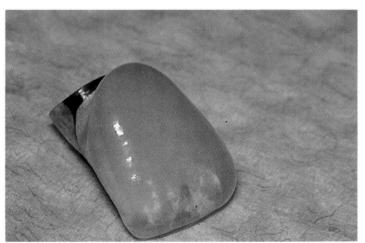

Fig. 5-163,A

Figure 5-163,B illustrates the porcelain fused to metal restoration as it seats over the abutment cylinder.

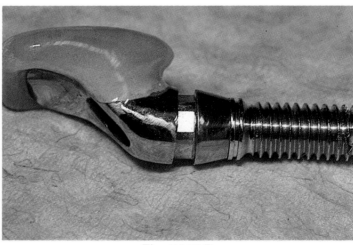

Fig. 5-163,B

When ready for delivery, cement is applied to the abutment cylinder (Fig. 5-164,A) and the porcelain-fused to metal restoration is positioned (Fig. 5-164,B).

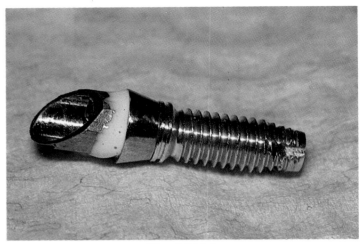

Fig. 5-164,A

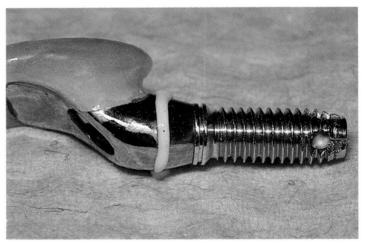

Fig. 5-164,B

Excess cement is removed, and the crown/abutment cylinder is now secured as one piece (Fig. 5-165,A).

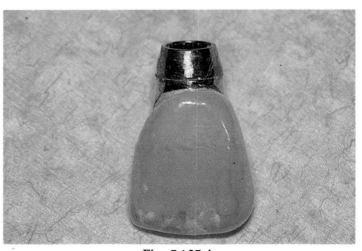

Fig. 5-165,A

The restoration connects to the implant fixture with a titanium screw (Fig. 5-165,B). The hexagon of the abutment cylinder must align properly with the implant hexagon in order to seat the restoration.

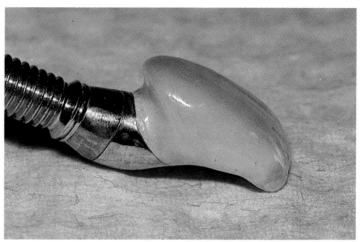

Fig. 5-165,B

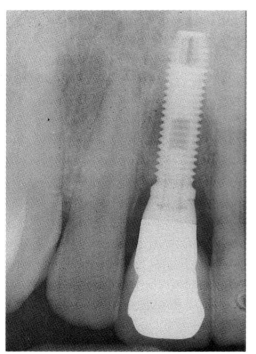

Fig. 5-166,A

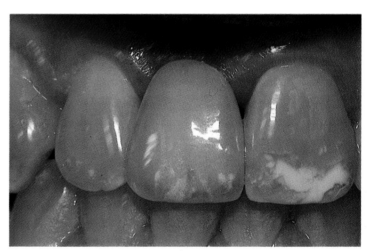

Fig. 5-166,B

Note the radiographs illustrating the connection of the crown, abutment cylinder, and implant fixture (Fig. 5-166,A). The restoration has been delivered in Figure 5-166,B.

REFERENCES

1. Johansson, C., Albrektsson, T.: Integration of screw implants in the rabbit: A one year followup of removal torque of titanium implants. Int. J. Oral & Max. Implants 2:2, 69-75, 1987.

PRODUCT CREDITS

1. Buffalo Dental Mfg. Co. Inc., Syosett, New York.

2. "UCLA" Abutments provided by Implant Support Systems, Irvine, Califoria.

CHAPTER 6   Complications

INTRODUCTION

At UCLA, the rate of complications has been quite low with the "Branemark" system. However, there are some complications which can be a significant, and more importantly, which indicate flaws associated with the design or fabrication of the implant-supported prosthesis.

COMPLICATIONS ASSOCIATED WITH SURGICAL PLACEMENT AND ABUTMENT CONNECTION

Dihiscence

Premature dihiscense of an implant may impair the process of osseointegration and in some instances require surgical intervention. Mucosal flaps are raised on either side of the exposed implant in question and closed appropriately. Such exposures are rare. They may occur due to a number of factors, including flap design and closure, local irritation from a removable prosthesis worn post surgically, or suture abscesses. Exposures occurring six weeks postsurgery or beyond need not be closed surgically. Clinical experience at UCLA has indicated that osseointegration occurs in almost all cases when the implant exposure occurs six weeks or more postsurgery. However, these implant exposures should be cleaned regularly, and use of chlorhexadine is a valuable means of maintaining low levels of plaque.

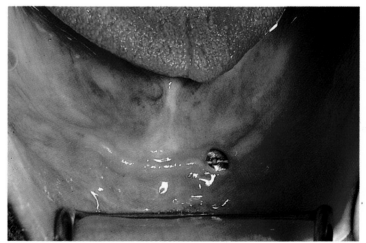

Fig. 6-1

This dihiscense occurred in a partially edentulous patient. In the posterior mandible of the partially edentulous patient, the muco-periosteum may be thin, and the risk of early implant exposure is greater than other sites. In this incidence, good oral hygiene was maintained around the exposure site and the implant fixture became osseointegrated.

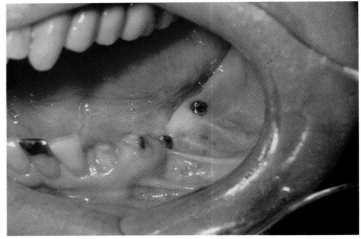

Fig. 6-2

Seating of Abutment Cylinder

During abutment connection, care must be taken to properly seat the abutment onto the implant fixture. Otherwise, both the abutment screw and the fixture will be at increased risk of fracture. In addition, the resultant gap may harbor microorganisms thereby predisposing to mucosal edema and granulation tissue formation, as seen in this patient. The abutment must be removed, the excess tissue excised, and the abutment cylinder resecured in position.

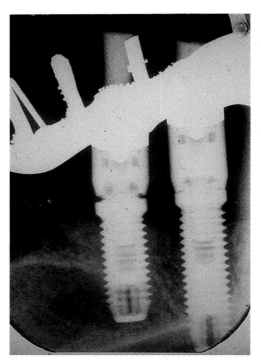

Fig. 6-3

Length of Abutment Cylinder

The top of this abutment is at the level of the mucosal margin. Ideally, the abutment cylinders must project 2-3 mm above the mucosal margin. If not, the mucosa is susceptible to inflammation with resulting edema, hypertrophy, and granulation tissue formation. The reasons for the above are now becoming evident. The interface between the gold cylinder and the abutment is not as precise as one would desire. Dental plaque accumulates in this interface in significant amounts. If this interface is close to the mucosal margin, an inflammatory response may result. Abutments which do not project an appropriate distance above the mucosa should be exchanged for longer ones.

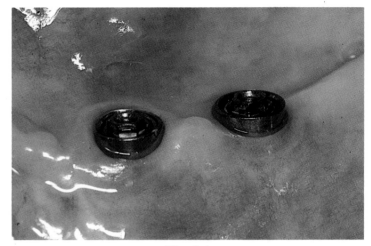

Fig. 6-4

This patient had been wearing a fixed bone-anchored bridge for six weeks. Note the accumulation of plaque on top of the abutment cylinders. Had the junction of the abutment and the gold cylinder (now incorporated within the permanent restoration) been in contact with the mucosa, inflammation may have resulted.

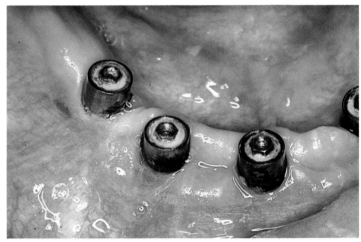

Fig. 6-5

A healing cap was used to facilitate oral hygiene when surgically induced edema (as a result of abutment connection) resulted in the mucosa level rising above the abutment cylinder. If, upon organization of the wound, the relationship between the mucosal level and the abutment cylinder is not appropriate, the abutment should be exchanged for a longer one.

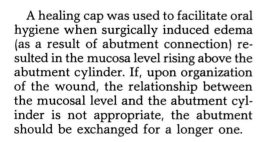

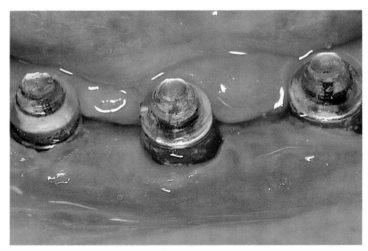

Fig. 6-6

This patient presented with significant mucosal hypertrophy after wearing her fixed bone-anchored bridge for six months. The perceived cause was plaque and calculus accumulation on the exposed surface of the abutment cylinder and the undersurface of the prosthesis. Resolution was obtained by means of a two-week course of antibiotics in combination with twice-daily applications of chlorhexidine. Equally important, the abutment cylinders did not project sufficiently above the mucosal margin. To eliminate recurrent gingival hypertrophy, the abutment cylinders should be exchanged for longer ones and the prosthesis remade.

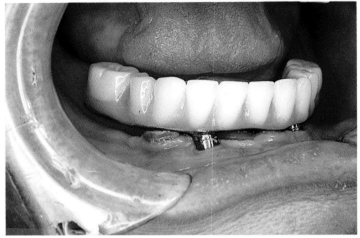

Fig. 6-7

Loose Abutment Cylinder

A loose abutment cylinder (shown here) not only mechanically irritates the mucosa, but also allows the excessive accumulation of microorganisms at the interface between the abutment and implant fixture. The resultant inflammatory response precipitated edema and granulation tissue.

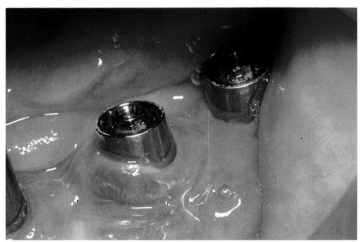

Fig. 6-8

Damaged Abutment Cylinder

Pure titanium is a soft metal; it is easily scratched or indented. In this patient (Fig. 6-9,A) premature occlusal contact has resulted in a deformation of the abutment cylinder.

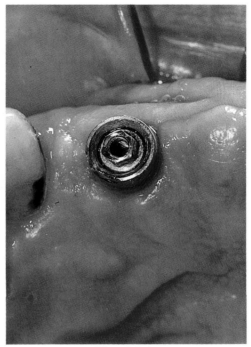

Fig. 6-9,A

In the next patient (Fig. 6-9,B) the metal framework from an old removable partial denture has likewise damaged the surface of the titanium abutment. In order to proceed with prosthesis fabrication, these damaged abutments must be replaced.

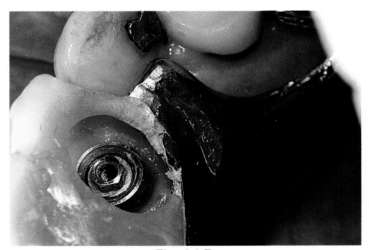

Fig. 6-9,B

Diabetes

It is well known that long-term diabetes results in compromise of oral mucous membranes. Although osseointegration has been successful and there are sufficient amounts of keratinized attached tissue adjacent to the abutment cylinder, inflammation, ulceration, and edema persisted indefinitely in this diabetic patient. Resolution was finally obtained with prolonged use of chlorhexidine.

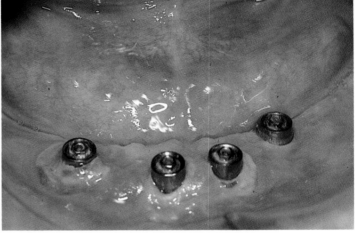

Fig. 6-10

Failure of a Fixture to Osseointegrate

Lack of osseointegration is usually detected immediately upon abutment connection or soon thereafter. This implant fixture became symptomatic almost immediately, although the discomfort was not severe. In this patient, a persistent purulent exudate was expressed from around the abutment cylinder, and within a few days the implant fixture was visably mobile. Such fixtures should be removed immediately and at least a six-month healing period allowed before one considers placing another implant at this particular site.

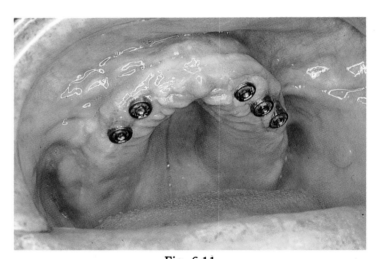

Fig. 6-11

In this patient the abutments had been connected to the implant fixtures ten days prior. Signs of infection are lacking but close examination reveals slight mobility of the two fixtures. In our experience, implant fixtures placed in the posterior maxillary quadrants where the quality of bone is poorest fail to osseointegrate at a rate higher than other oral sites.

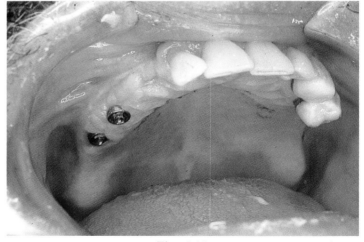

Fig. 6-12

Implant fixtures lacking osseointegration are easily removed. Upon fixture removal, the soft-tissue lining at the site should be removed carefully by curettage in order to promote filling of this defect with normal bone.

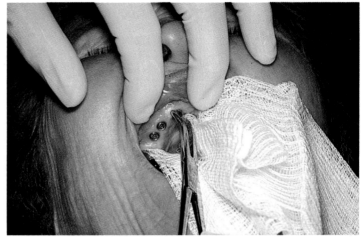

Fig. 6-13

Implant Related Infection

This is a fistula associated with an implant fixture. Neither a course of antibiotics (per oral & IV) based on culture and sensitivity nor surgical debridement of the infected site resolved the infection. It is the only Branemark-type mandibular fixture placed by the UCLA team that has been removed to date. It is believed that the infection was precipitated by the formation of a subperiosteal hematoma resulting from perforation of the inferior border. The active organism cultured has often been implicated in infections associated with hip implants. Antibiotic choice was limited because of the patient's allergy to many of the more widely used and effective antimicrobial drugs.

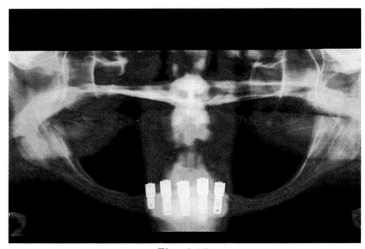

Fig. 6-14

A panoramic radiograph of the previous patient indicated significant bone loss associated with the centrally positioned implant fixture. Since the mandible was thin buccal-lingually, further bone loss could have led to pathologic fracture of the mandible. The fixture was consequently removed.

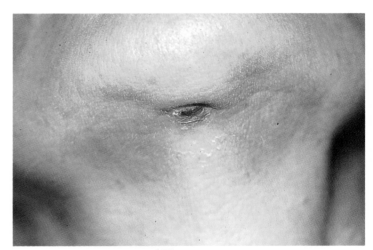

Fig. 6-15

A specially designed trephine instrument (Fig. 6-16,A) was used to remove this osseointegrated, but infected implant fixture.

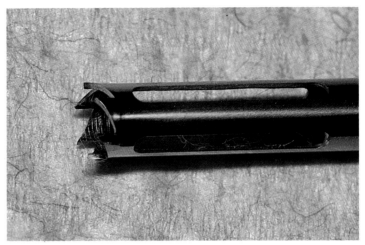

Fig. 6-16,A

Histologic analysis of the specimen (Fig. 6-26,B) revealed the top two thirds of the implant fixture to be osseointegrated.

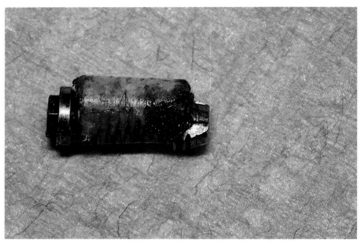

Fig. 6-16,B

Malpositioned Implant Fixtures

On occasion, implant fixtures which appear to be osseointegrated can not be used to support a definitive prosthesis. As one can see from this panoramic radiograph, the angulation of this implant fixture was not compatible with the adjacent implants and therefore it was buried permanently beneath the mucosa.

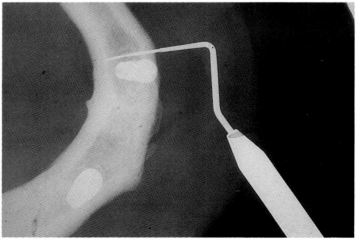

Fig. 6-17

In this patient, because of the maxilla's poor bone quality, extra fixtures were placed. Upon uncovering, it was clear that all fixtures were osseointegrated. An overdenture was planned and it was felt advantageous to use only four of the six implants. The remaining two were left buried beneath the oral mucosa and stand in reserve.

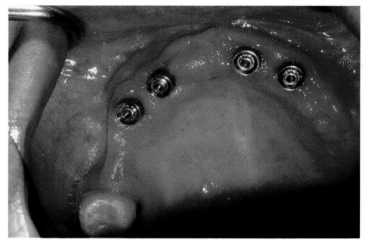

Fig. 6-18

FRACTURE OF COMPONENTS

Fracture of Hardware: Almost all hardware elements are susceptible to fracture. Fractures can be indicative of a number of problems.

    a.   A manufacturing imperfection associated with the particular hardware component.
    b.   A discrepancy in adaptation of the dental restoration to the abutment cylinders.
    c.   Inappropriate occlusal loads applied during function.
    d.   Occlusal prematurities.
    e.   Bruxism and clenching by the patient.
    f.   Excessive bone resorption around implant fixtures.
    g.   Significant occlusal loads applied to malposed implants.

Any failure of hardware should prompt the clinician to carefully scrutinize the occlusion, precision of fit of the restoration, and the bone levels around the implant fixture.

Fig. 6-19

Gold Screw Fracture

The first element to fail is generally the gold alloy screw used to secure the dental restoration to the abutment cylinder. As mentioned previously, such failures require that the occlusion be evaluated carefully and the metal framework interfacing with the abutments checked for accuracy of adaptation. This patient was a persistent bruxer and has broken two gold screws. After the second episode, the fixed bone-anchored bridge was exchanged for an overdenture. Removal of fractured gold screws can be accomplished by either a slow-speed contra-angle (by reversing the rotation) or a small dental instrument such as a scaler or dental explorer. A simpler method would be to remove and exchange the abutment screw for a new abutment screw and gold alloy screw.

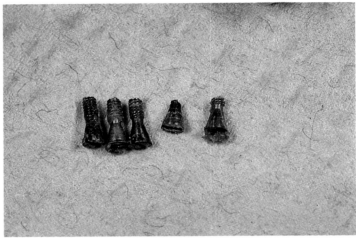

Fig. 6-20

Abutment Screw Fracture

An abutment screw fractured in this patient. Such fractures are often associated with ill-fitting components or occlusal discrepancies, and may be accompanied by bone loss. Perapical radiographs and a thorough analysis of the restoration are indicated. In this patient moderate bone loss was seen around the implant fixture.

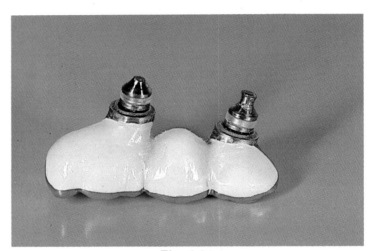

Fig. 6-21

Fractured abutment screws are retrieved easily. In this patient, a small round bur was embedded on top of the fractured abutment screw with a slow-speed contra-angle. The screw was removed by reversing the rotation of the dental handpiece. A sharply pointed dental instrument can also be used to facilitate removal. This method may be preferred when removing screws from implant fixtures where access is difficult, in order to avoid damaging the threads on the inner surface of the implant fixture.

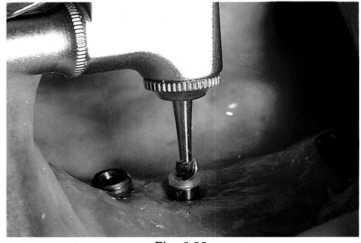

Fig. 6-22

Implant Fixture Fracture

Fractured fixtures are more difficult to retrieve (Figs. 6-23,A and B). If removal is indicated, the rotary trephine instrument (demonstrated previously) must be used. Fractured fixtures are often seen in association with rapid crestal bone loss. The usual causative factor is inappropriate occlusal stress. If the fracture occurs below the level of the abutment screw, the entire fixture should be removed. If sufficient threads for the abutment screw remain, the top of the fixture can be leveled and a longer abutment cylinder then secured to the implant fixture.

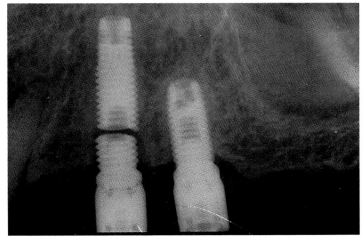

Fig. 6-23,A

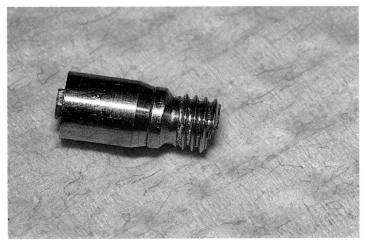

Fig. 6-23,B

Metal Framework For Dental Restoration

On occasion overdenture or fixed bone-anchored bridge frameworks will fracture (Figs. 6-24,A and B). The most common fracture site is the area just distal to the terminal implant fixture. Most such fractures are caused either by inadequate bulk in this region or by voids or discrepancies formed during casting.

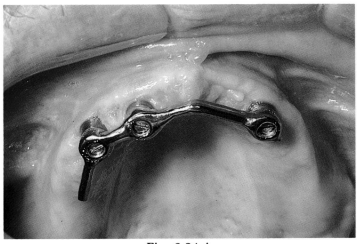

Fig. 6-24,A

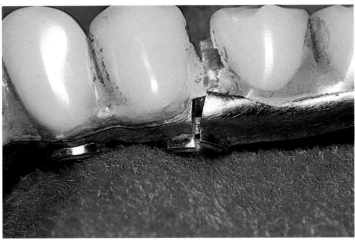

Fig. 6-24,B

POOR ORAL HYGIENE

Poor oral hygiene results in accumulation of plaque and calculus, which lead to mucosal inflammation. The patient must be well-educated regarding the appropriate oral hygiene techniques and should be followed by the dental hygienest four times annually. Overdenture bars are not immune to these oral accumulations. If hygiene is not appropriate, mucosal hypertrophy will be the inevitable result.

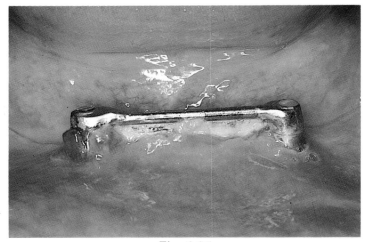

Fig. 6-25

Calculus adheres tenaciously to the machined titanium surfaces and is quite difficult to remove. Such accumulation are unavoidable in some patients and close follow-up is mandatory.

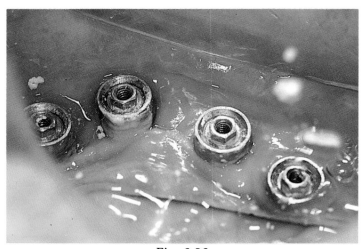

Fig. 6-26